# Stretched to the Limits

*of related interest*

**Supporting Autistic People through Pregnancy and Childbirth**
*Hayley Morgan, Emma Durman and Karen Henry*
ISBN 978 1 83997 105 1
eISBN 978 1 83997 106 8

**Supporting Survivors of Sexual Abuse**
**Through Pregnancy and Childbirth**
**A Guide for Midwives, Doulas and Other Healthcare Professionals**
*Kicki Hansard*
*Forewords by Penny Simkin and Phyllis Klaus*
ISBN 978 1 84819 424 3
eISBN 978 0 85701 377 4

**Supporting Queer Birth**
**A Book for Birth Professionals and Parents**
*AJ Silver*
ISBN 978 1 83997 045 0
eISBN 978 1 83997 046 7

**Supporting Fat Birth**
**Supporting Body Positive Birth**
*AJ Silver*
ISBN 978 1 83997 633 9
eISBN 978 1 83997 634 6

# STRETCHED to the Limits

*Supporting Women with Hypermobile
Ehlers-Danlos Syndrome (hEDS) Through
Pregnancy, Labour, and Postnatally*

## Rachel Fitz-Desorgher

*Foreword by Susan Booth and Sarah Hamilton*

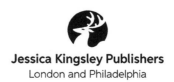

**Jessica Kingsley Publishers**
London and Philadelphia

First published in Great Britain in 2024 by Jessica Kingsley Publishers
An imprint of John Murray Press

1

Copyright © Rachel Fitz-Desorgher 2024

Foreword copyright © Susan Booth and Sarah Hamilton 2024

Front cover image source: Shutterstock®.

Disclaimer: The information contained in this book is not intended to replace the services of trained medical professionals or to be a substitute for medical advice. You are advised to consult a doctor on any matters relating to your health, and in particular on any matters that may require diagnosis or medical attention.

A CIP catalogue record for this title is available from the British Library and the Library of Congress

ISBN 978 1 83997 249 2
eISBN 978 1 83997 250 8

Printed and bound by CPI Group (UK) Ltd, Croydon, CR0 4YY

Jessica Kingsley Publishers' policy is to use papers that are natural, renewable and recyclable products and made from wood grown in sustainable forests. The logging and manufacturing processes are expected to conform to the environmental regulations of the country of origin.

Jessica Kingsley Publishers
Carmelite House
50 Victoria Embankment
London EC4Y 0DZ

www.jkp.com

John Murray Press
Part of Hodder & Stoughton Ltd
An Hachette Company

*For my mum, Pam, who devoted her life to empowering women to birth with confidence and for whom I wish my book had come sooner.*

# Acknowledgements

Bringing this book to you has required the skills and support of a team to whom I am totally indebted and who should now come out of the shadows to take their well-earned thanks.

First, my commissioning editor, Carole, who stayed calm and encouraging throughout, soothing my anxieties, enduring my chunterings and, along with the rest of the team (Rosa, Masooma, Judy, Vicki and Jenny), eased my manuscript into shape whilst beautifully preserving my voice.

The staff at Nirvana Spa who kept me going through my very hardest writing months with endless cups of coffee and a welcoming pool, and Sue who skilfully played the piano so I could relax and sing.

My readers, Gemma, Karen, Linda and Lorna, who gave up their time to read my manuscript, and the army of amazing mums, credited next to their quotes, who generously shared their stories – at last, your voices will be heard. My treasured midwife friends, 'The Mitzies': Jennie, Jules and Linda, who continue to uplift and inspire me.

My sister, Charlotte who always knows when to tell me I'm amazing and also when I'm an idiot – that is what sisters are for and I have the very best!

Heartfelt thanks to Ollie – your beautiful photos (thank you Lauren, Lynsey and Malika and your gorgeous babies) shine out of these pages, and Amy for introducing us and making the photoshoot such a lovely experience.

My talented son, Alasdair, who found time to draw the illustrations whilst already being up to his neck in work, creating the simplicity and clarity which I just couldn't source elsewhere.

Finally, my men! My husband, Tim, and my sons, Ted, Alasdair, Laurence and Connor, for the joy, love and support you always give me. Tim, my beloved soulmate – you are my rock, against which I know I can always lean.

# Contents

# Part II: EDS and Pregnancy

# Part III: EDS and Labour

# Part IV: Postnatal

# Foreword

With hypermobile Ehlers-Danlos Syndrome (hEDS), knowledge is key – not only for patients but also, and especially, for professionals. *Stretched to the Limits* covers it all in the most insightful and educational way. Ehlers-Danlos Support UK was delighted to hear about Rachel's new book and the wealth of knowledge it will bring to professionals. Covering the patient from head to toe and inside out, *Stretched to the Limits* has it all and more.

Rachel has personal experience as a hEDS mother herself and this, along with her professional career in midwifery, makes her the perfect person to write a book for birthing professionals. The wealth of information and advice in this book will help keep hEDS women safer physically and emotionally. Members of Ehlers-Danlos Support UK's team have been guided through their pregnancy by Rachel, as have many members of the community, so being able to recommend this book is a joy. Rachel's passion for these mothers is visible throughout, and her ability to share not only her knowledge but her enthusiasm on the subject makes for a delightful read.

We've worked with Rachel for many years; her ability to connect deeply with the community has shone through and her expertise has been invaluable. From birthing plans to webinars, books and groups, Rachel's knowledge is limitless and this fantastic new book doesn't fall shy. We've referred many a mum through Rachel and it's always a delight to hear about the amazing insight she has shared not only with them but with the professionals involved in their pregnancy and birth.

There's a huge gap in knowledge around pregnancy and hypermobile Ehlers-Danlos Syndrome and Rachel has managed to fill that gap with this book. For those professionals desperate to help their patients, here is the book you need. We're thoroughly looking forward to recommending this book to many a birthing professional and to those women going through the mothering journey to share with their practitioners. The ability to impart this level of knowledge in such a calm, direct and evidence-based way is a skill, and one that Rachel most definitely possesses and demonstrates throughout.

From start to finish, outlining the condition itself to every step of pregnancy and postnatal needs, it covers everything a professional needs to know to best care for the expecting, birthing and postnatal hEDS mum. This book is a wonderful insight into the real experiences of patients, as well as providing scientific, evidence-based information to guide practice for birthing professionals. The information out there on hEDS can be difficult to navigate, but there is no need to worry any longer with the publication of *Stretched to the Limits*! There isn't a topic missed, no area of the body not covered and no question unanswered.

Rachel's honest, open and real-lived experiences create an easy read for busy professionals in a fast-paced environment. Understanding a multi-systemic condition is complex but everything is covered here: from subluxations to stress incontinence and birth plans to stitches.

With the joy of having a child comes anxiety and worry, and adding hypermobile Ehlers-Danlos Syndrome to that, which is likely to have further impact, can create a concoction of concern and anxiety; professionals with this book in their armour will not only instill confidence in their patients but also be able to demonstrate their in-depth knowledge and support these mothers in the best ways possible.

Whether you're new to hypermobile Ehlers-Danlos Syndrome or already familiar with it, *Stretched to the Limits* is a must-have for the professional's bookshelf. Rachel's awareness of the true nature of hypermobile Ehlers-Danlos Syndrome and its impact on pregnancy and birth is exceptional. What a delight to be able to share this knowledge and experience with others!

*Susan Booth and Sarah Hamilton*
*Ehlers-Danlos Support UK*

# Introduction

## *Who Am I?*

This book is the book I wish I'd had for myself in my decades as a practising midwife. It is the book I wish I'd had to share with my midwives and birth supporters when I was pregnant with my four sons and it is the book I am proud to be able to share with you and your clients now.

I am a woman with hypermobile Ehlers-Danlos syndrome (hEDS), I am a busy mum and grand-mum and, despite retiring from the midwifery part of my working life a couple of years ago, I am a midwife to my very bones. I am *you*! I understand your drive, your commitment and your passion and I understand the pressures you are under to keep your woman safe, at the same time as empowering her to self-advocate. I really know how much you want to practise your considerable skills at protecting normality – to give your woman the experience she wants and that will ease her into her new journey as a mother in the gentlest and most life-affirming way possible. It is my genuine desire to give you the knowledge and confidence you need to use those skills whenever you are supporting a woman with hEDS.

As you will discover in these pages, the term 'Ehlers-Danlos syndrome' actually covers 13 individual genetic conditions affecting the body's connective tissue. The subtypes have some symptoms in common but also many impacts that are unique to that subtype. The most common of these subtypes, and the focus of this book, is the hypermobile type (hEDS). There is a big overlap in signs and symptoms between the subtypes, and also some divergences, and I will highlight these as we go along. But, unless I flag up otherwise, we are talking about hEDS.

Now, as a midwife or doula, you will almost certainly have come across women with hEDS during your career and will definitely have supported many who are affected by less profound connective tissue conditions, such as hypermobility spectrum disorder (HSD), who can present with at least some of the same challenges for pregnancy, labour and birth as those with hEDS.

Many women start their parenting journey undiagnosed, and those that do have a clinical diagnosis often experience being treated as if they have a different Ehlers-Danlos syndrome (EDS) subtype with different implications for care. Imagine that you were a woman in an uncomplicated twin pregnancy, with carers who only knew about conjoined twin pregnancy and so treated you as if you and your babies were at the same very high risk of complications as if your babies were conjoined. Imagine how confused, scared and unseen you might feel as you found yourself on a care pathway that simply wasn't appropriate for you and which could lead you down that 'slippery slope of intervention' that we, as midwives, try to avoid.

This is the sort of experience that women with hEDS face – they give a diagnosis of hEDS at booking and their midwife, being none the wiser, packs them off to see a consultant who duly starts them on a care pathway designed for women with the rather different classic EDS (cEDS) with its increased risk of premature birth. One mum I spoke to had even been treated by a consultant who, it appears, muddled her subtype with vascular EDS (vEDS) with its risk of uterine and blood vessel rupture! As you might imagine, this poor, bemused mum took quite a bit of talking down as I helped her have a less terrifying and more realistic picture of how her pregnancy and birth could pan out.

Paradoxically, because of the tissue-softening nature of hEDS, along with other effects of the condition, far from presenting midwives with a high-risk birth experience to manage, women with hEDS often labour and birth very swiftly and so can potentially provide midwives and doulas with the opportunity to practise in a very holistic, drug-free and low-tech way, to use their core skills and to maybe learn some new ones. As you will see, supporting women with hEDS towards a calm, low-tech, midwife-led experience can reduce the impact, on very many, of the myriad effects on their physical and mental well-being and, in turn, give you the 'with woman' experience that brings tremendous job satisfaction.

This book is aimed at you as a skilled, highly trained and evidence-based professional, and you will find the evidence referenced throughout, as you would expect. I will help you appreciate how often this evidence lumps various subtypes of EDS together, resulting in women being led down a path that could, potentially, cause the very complications you are trying to avoid, creating a self-fulfilling prophesy.

Chapter by chapter, we will take a look at the various ways that hEDS can affect the various bodily systems and the implications for pregnancy, labour, birth and postnatally. We will look at how, by working with rather than against the hEDS body and mind, you can keep your woman safer physically and emotionally – wherever possible providing her with midwife-led care, whilst also ensuring that you know when it's appropriate to transfer to consultant-led care.

Ultimately, I want the voices of the women themselves to shine through and to speak to you of their lived experience and what they want and need to feel safe in their complex, quirky bodies so that they can birth their babies confidently and safely. So I will be drawing on my own experiences as a midwife and a woman with hEDS as well as on those of many others who have generously offered to give their stories, in the hope that your future clients can benefit and thrive under your expert care.

I want this book to be easy to read, otherwise...you won't read it! So expect a rather different type of educational book from the somewhat dry, dense and cold tome you might be used to. I hope that this book speaks to you, draws you in and reminds you of why you became a midwife in the first place – to truly walk with your woman, wherever and however she is in her world, to advocate for her whilst also empowering her to advocate for herself and to support her to make informed choices and decisions about herself, her body and her baby.

Enjoy the journey!

# PART I

# A Guided Tour of the EDS Body

## CHAPTER 1

# The Skin

## Introduction

It would be easy to dive straight into your comfort zones: to get stuck into the nitty gritty of caring for a newly pregnant woman with hEDS. However, I want to take this slowly and help you get a real understanding of the condition first, outside of your sphere of knowledge, and then look at it in the context of your practice. So in this first part of the book we shall look at each system in turn and in detail to see how it affects the normal working of the body, and only then will we hunker down and consider how each stage of the pregnancy-to-mothering journey might be affected and what you might need to consider when caring for your hEDS client.

There are many common co-morbidities associated with hEDS, and I will draw your attention briefly to these where appropriate whilst keeping the main focus on the core features and symptoms of the syndrome.

Let's start with considering the absolute basics of what EDS is, and then we will start on our hEDS grand tour.

## What Is EDS?

The Ehlers-Danlos syndromes consist of a group of heritable connective tissue disorders characterised by joint hypermobility, skin hyper-extensibility or elasticity, and skin fragility. There has been debate over the decades about how many subtypes there are and how to classify them, given the potentially subjective measures of skin stretchiness and how soft the skin is. After all, babies have softer skin and the elderly have thinner and stretchier skin, and there are endless variabilities in between those stages of life and between two individuals. And so, in 2017, the

International EDS Consortium proposed a new classification system recognising 13 distinct subtypes.[1] The vast majority of these subtypes are extremely rare and some, like vascular (vEDS) and kyphoscoliotic (kEDS), can be life-shortening.

Of the 13 EDS subtypes, the hypermobility type (hEDS) is the most common, but population prevalence is tricky to estimate due to the ongoing confusion over clinical diagnosis and the overlap in so many symptoms between hEDS and the more common hypermobility spectrum disorder.[2] In addition, many women, traipsing back and forth to their doctor, get treated issue by issue without anyone ever joining the hEDS dots. To give you an idea of how far we are from nailing the prevalence debate, the figures given vary from 1:500 as quoted in a Welsh study[3] to anywhere up to 1:20,000.[4]

EDS is not the only group of syndromes affecting the connective tissue, but are on the same continuum as others such as Loeys-Dietz syndrome and Marfans syndrome. Because of the common thread between all these conditions – namely faulty connective tissue – there is quite a crossover in signs and symptoms, further adding to the confusion with diagnosis.

Given this lack of clarity, in terms of your practice, when faced with a woman who seems to be a shoe-in for everything you will learn in these pages, even if she doesn't have a formal diagnosis, it would be wise to at least consider the possibility that she might have hEDS and prepare accordingly. In short, if it looks like a duck and walks like a duck and quacks like a duck, then you'd be wise to care for it like it's a duck unless it whips off its cute duck disguise and announces that it's actually a cat! Better to be safe than sorry when it comes to supporting a pregnant or labouring woman.

## A Word of Warning – the Me Too Issue!

Living with hEDS can be exhausting – chronic pain, sleep disturbances, trips to physios...and all our mates asking if they might have hEDS too! It goes something like this: someone asks me what hEDS is and I try to give a potted version, which leads to the follow-up question of how it affects me. So I might mention my very visible hypermobility and then...'Oh! I'm flexible – maybe I have EDS!' Or I mention my easy bruising and 'Yes! Me too! I get bruises and have *no* idea how I got them – have you tried taking vitamin C?' and then they spot my ever-present hot water bottle along with my bare feet and that really puts the cat amongst the pigeons: 'I am so much colder than my husband but you haven't got any socks on. No wonder you need a hot water bottle! Have you tried wearing an extra jumper and thick socks?' And so it goes on. No doubt, as you make your way through this book, at some point you will probably decide you've got hEDS. What marks out hEDS from just the general all-glitches-welcome brand of humankind is the sheer array and severity of what might otherwise be normal stuff, alongside some truly weird stuff. There is collagen everywhere and simply hundreds of gene mutations giving rise to a continuum of degrees of bendiness and tendency to bruise. As a tribe, women are more flexible than men, feel colder, bruise more easily and often sleep a little differently, especially at key hormonal stages in their life. With hEDS there is more, much, much more. When a woman with hEDS is trying to explain her lived experience to you, try hard not to rush in to 'Ooh yes, me too!' It can make our experience feel misunderstood, diminished and as if we are seen as being simply a bit more wimpy than everyone else.

## hEDS in Particular

hEDS, like its other family subtypes, is most often characterised by the visible skin and joint symptoms, but the tendrils put out by this syndrome reach into every nook and cranny of the body due to the sheer abundance of collagen and connective tissue throughout. This results in a multi-system condition which can impact every organ in the body, including the brain, and the nervous and immune systems, as we shall see. Let's start by considering the villain in all this – faulty collagen...

## What Are Collagen and Connective Tissue?

Collagen is, quite simply, the most abundant protein in the human body, comprising 28 types,[5] and is found everywhere from muscles and tendons through to teeth and placental tissue.[6] Type 1 is the single most prevalent collagen, being a component in bones, tendons and muscles, and this type alone has some 300 mutations giving rise to various connective tissue disorders.[7] Whilst the rarer EDS subtypes have had their affected genes mapped, this is not the case yet for hEDS, and so diagnosis is made clinically through history-taking of signs and symptoms[8] along with the use of the new 2017 diagnostic criteria.[9]

## The EDS Skin

Let's start with the largest body organ of all, the skin. The first time I palpated the pregnant belly of a woman with hEDS I almost jumped! Until that moment I had no idea what my husband meant when he spoke about the texture of my skin – your own skin felt through your own fingertips feels somewhat different from how it feels to someone else, it seems. The hEDS skin feels silky smooth and unusually yielding. The softness is not the everyday softness of freshly shaved and oiled flesh – it feels…well, just unbelievably and unusually soft. Enough for people to remark on it again and again. The faulty collagen means that there is a lack of strength to the fibre and so fingers can sink into flesh with little resistance. The few times I've submitted myself to the bruising experience of a massage, I get the same reaction of surprise from the masseuse.

> *Despite having extremely veiny, thin, fragile, allergy-prone skin that bruises easily, somehow I manage to look very young for my age!?*
>
> Omi

On the fleshy thighs of a woman, the much-described 'dough-like' flesh is particularly noticeable. Imagine a couple of pairs of tights. One pair is super-soft and maybe a little old. The other pair is designed for maximum support, maybe even TED stockings. Now imagine taking a large bucket of marbles and pouring some into the legs of each pair. The soft tights would fail to shape the marbles at all, they'd prolapse out with nothing to hold them firmly in place creating a very lumpy surface. The support tights would hold the marbles so firmly that you might not be able to discern each individual marble under the surface. Needless to say I have had to accept that, despite having swum like a demon regularly since babyhood, every fleshy area on my body looks like that saggy pair of tights with a lack of sleek taut support over the underlying knobbly bits. I have a photo of myself as a young student nurse on holiday in Corfu with my mates. We are all sat down on a table top grinning for the camera, our thighs on full display, and mine are just sprawling out! And I was the skinny one.

You will read a lot about the skin hyper-extensibility in EDS. Those with classic type (cEDS) tend to have very much more marked stretchiness compared to those with hEDS but, with so many genes involved, there can be a lot of crossover of symptoms and so your hEDS client might have super-stretchy skin (see Figure 1.1). It is often described as being less prone to fine age-related wrinkles due to being so stretchy, but also prone to stretch marks due to its fragility. Sounds like a paradox, I know. It can be rather thin, often most noticeably on the hands, where the veins look particularly prominent, bulging up, unconstrained by the soft skin. This super-stretchy but rather thin skin can be a 'good-thing-bad-thing' in the birthing room as, we will explore in Part III.

> *Certain types of stitches and stitching methods seem to not work with me either – the wound will just come undone and open up.*
>
> Gee

As well as being more fragile, the skin can be slower to heal. This skin fragility and slowness to heal is more marked in cEDS but often also present to a lesser degree in hEDS, so you might notice some odd scars called hypertrophic scars. They are wider and more wrinkly than regular scars and can appear from even the slightest bit of damage. Again, these scars (also known as cigarette paper scars due to their appearance) are much more prevalent and obvious in cEDS,[10] but you might notice them on the body of your hEDS client too.

> *The damage a plaster can do after a blood test is worse than the needle mark itself.*
>
> Emily

The thinner skin is prone to letting the blood vessels underneath show through and this is often most noticeable around the eyes, with dark rings a feature of even the best-rested woman. As it happens, hEDS can really mess with sleep but, nonetheless, those dark bags are just as likely her au naturel look. An ex-boyfriend once told me I had eyes like a bear. Big and beautiful? No, deep set with dark bags! I repeat...he's an ex!

The skin hair, if present, is often extremely soft and downy – a bit like baby hair – because of the faulty hEDS collagen, and the head hair also tends to be extremely soft and more likely to break with normal brushing. Remember this fragile hair on fragile skin if you're taking a razor to it! On the other hand, if you're waiting to use the hairdryer after a swim, cross fingers the lass in front has hEDS – she'll be done in the twinkling of an eye! Me? Takes me an average of 20 seconds to dry my sparse, baby-fine hair after a dip and I'm very intolerant of anyone ahead of me in the hairdryer queue who is blessed with a thick, strong head of hair and needs to hog the dryer for half the morning! For some of us, the hair is so fine and fragile that we also have very sparse body hair, which saves us a small fortune in trips to the waxing salon!

The finger and toe nails can also be very fragile and there is an increased tendency for ingrown toenails.[11] This, along with the ability of the feet to blister even in long-loved shoes, can make footwear and foot care a real problem, which is not improved by the extra weight burden of pregnancy. Also, whilst we are down in the foot area, you might spot some round, soft, pale lumps of flesh around the heels and sides of the feet. These are piezogenic pedal papules: benign herniations of elastic tissue and subcutaneous fat that break through the dermis when the foot is put under pressure such as when standing; although generally painless and of no consequence, they can cause pain in some people, making standing and walking uncomfortable. These little lumps are seen in greater numbers in a person with EDS than in a less stretchy-skinned individual[12] and can also appear on the heel of the hands when the palm is pressed.

Finally, you will almost certainly spot bruises. A lot of bruises.[13] I have had to reassure fellow swimmers at the poolside and my poor bloke has had to endure some pretty fierce looks when he takes to the water with me. My midwife-masseuse mate refuses to massage me now as I ping up bruises whilst she pummels. Massage leg oedema a little enthusiastically at one antenatal visit and you might see the dark blue-green witnesses the following visit. Advise your hEDS client to use her knuckles to relieve breast engorgement and you could be submitting her to painful bruises for the next few weeks. For kinder tips, see Chapter 17. Of course, you will still need to screen for domestic abuse during your professional relationship with your hEDS client but be aware that she really might have sustained all those bruises from the mildest of knocks. You will learn more about the vascular system in Chapter 3.

**Note:** Babies and toddlers sporting the hEDS genes may have even more bruises than their non-hEDS playmates,[14] so sensitive questioning and awareness is vital in health care and educational settings. Nursery staff need to be made aware that even holding the legs during a poon-ami nappy change might result in bruising, which can be alarming for anyone not prepared.

In summary, the hEDS skin, lacking as it does the usual support and strength of regular collagen, tends to be unusually soft, yielding to the touch, stretchy, fine and thin. The skin tends to break more easily, heal more slowly and scar unusually, and the hair and nails are also often soft and fragile. Bruising can be caused by minimal trauma and be visible for longer due to the thin nature of the overlying skin.

Beauty may only be skin deep; hEDS travels a lot further in, as we shall see...

*Sometimes though it feels like my skin is so sensitive I can't bear to be touched.*

Lauren

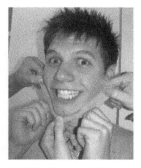

*Figure 1.1 Your hEDS client might have super-stretchy skin. The author's super-stretchy son!*

## CHAPTER 2

# The Musculoskeletal System

## Introduction

There are 206 bones, 600 muscles, approximately 900 ligaments and about 4000 tendons in the human musculoskeletal system. On top of this there is cartilage and connective tissue, and the whole lot works together to keep us upright, stable, moving, and aware of our movement through space. The bones are held in correct alignment by the muscles, tendons and ligaments, and cushioned by the cartilage. It is the normal structure of the connective tissues throughout the musculoskeletal system that provides that stability and support, and helps to prevent injuries such as sprains and dislocations. The musculoskeletal system also provides protection for the vital organs such as the lungs, liver and heart.[1] With this many different elements, just imagine the range of problems that could arise in the musculoskeletal system from a fault in the connective tissue!

Joint flexibility is the 'shop window' of hEDS and the thing that most of us will demonstrate as we attempt to describe our condition. People look admiringly at our ability to touch our toes with astonishing ease and then assume that this must make movement comfortable, graceful and easy. Surely we glide effortlessly through the world, our limber limbs bending quickly around obstacles as we dash off to our next advanced yoga class? Nothing could be further from the truth: for smooth, safe and lithe movement in space there needs to be just the right amount of tension in the musculoskeletal system. People with hEDS have just the wrong amount!

*I used to entertain my friends by sitting in the lotus position and wrapping my feet above my head long before gym-style yoga caught on!*

Joey

When starting out on the long road to a clinical diagnosis, the first test that is often carried out is called the Beighton score.[2] This possibly over-simplistic check is a quick, rough and ready way of seeing just how obviously bendy someone is. Only certain joints are checked for flexibility (little fingers, wrists, elbows, knees, spine) and a score then given out of 9; the higher the score, the more flexible the patient. A high score is obviously indicative of hypermobility but, for some with hEDS, the more obvious joints are relatively normal whilst other, unchecked joints like the shoulders, jaw and ankles might be very affected. Affected boys, lacking the softening impact of progesterone, are often under-diagnosed simply because they score low. Their recurrent injuries and clumsiness might be put down to them being 'a typical boy' and so they fly under the hEDS radar. However, although by no means the only system of concern, as the effects on the musculoskeletal system are the most visible manifestation of hEDS, let's check through bit by bit to see what impacts your client might have experienced in life.

## Skeleton

To start with, let's consider the actual skeleton. As part of the whole big family of connective tissue disorders, many with hEDS share physical characteristics with other syndromes and, in particular, Marfans. When history-taking to form a diagnosis of hEDS, physicians will look for a 'Marfan habitus'.[3] Marfans causes visible impacts to the skeleton and, whilst not all hEDSers will present with Marfan habitus, many do to one extent or another, and it is important to remember that, even if your hEDS client does possess some of the following Marfan skeletal traits, they do not have the condition itself. Long limbs with a much bigger than average arm span are common – if a typical non-affected individual stands against a wall with arms outstretched to the side, the measurement from the end of one middle finger to the other will be less than or equal to their height. In those with Marfan habitus, that span is more than their height. Ask an hEDSer (let's sometimes use that term we use for ourselves) about their home-knit jumpers growing up and you will often be told that Nan always had to knit a couple of inches more on the arms! My own mum used to sigh when she was knitting for me and say, 'Well, of course, sweetheart, you are obviously *very* closely related to an orangutan!' and, in my own household, whenever my youngest son was showing us just how big something was, as he swung out his arms, we'd all duck.

On the end of those long arms you will often find long, tapered fingers which, combined with the extra-loose connections between the joints, give rise to another neat Marfanoid trick: the Steinberg sign. Here the extra-long fingers (arachnodactyly) enable the owner to grasp the opposite wrist to encircle it with the little finger and thumb so easily that the thumb tip covers the nail of the little finger. It doesn't serve any useful purpose except to impress friends in the pub – when they say 'you must have really skinny wrists' we can challenge them to have a go with their fingers on our wrists only to confound them when they can't get their own fingers anywhere close. Reaching into small, deep spaces to retrieve lost objects is also a great skill for those with arachnodactyly!

The jaw can be narrow and the teeth crowded, so a history of teeth extractions and orthodontic braces in childhood is common. The palate is often described as a 'church roof' palate because it is unusually high and narrow, and the mum with a baby with hEDS might well need extra help to get the hang of feeding in a particular way to avoid her nipples getting caught in and shredded by the exceptionally raised bony palate (see Chapter 17). The loose connections around the jaw allow for unusually large movement and so there might well be a history of temporomandibular joint dysfunction (TMJD) causing clicking and pain when talking or eating. And the jaw might lock or dislocate more easily – important to know for any future potential intubation.

The rib cage in Marfan habitus is often mis-shaped so that the lower ribs splay out and the sternum caves in (pectus excavatum) or out (pectus carinatum). In Marfans the former deformity can be severe and impact on heart and lung function, but in hEDS it tends to be obvious but much milder and, although the ribs might cause little indentations on the heart where they cave in, there is unlikely to be any associated pathology in function as a result. There are often heartbeat irregularities in hEDS but these are as a result of dysfunction of the autonomic nervous system (ANS), as we will see later, and not due to the unusual rib formation.

Like the arms, the legs might well be long and lanky, ending with long feet and toes. Look at those feet and you might notice a condition called 'sandal toe' (hallux varus) where there is a gap between the big and second toe making it look as if flip-flops have been worn for too long. This deformity can be acquired but is more likely to be congenital where there is a connective tissue disorder.[4] These long feet can also be very flat due to the lack of support from the connecting tissues, so buying shoes is generally a real trial. To give you an idea – when I sit down to have my feet measured in a shop, with my feet held off the ground, I come up as a size 5.5. When I stand I'm a 6.5 and then, once I've been walking around for an hour or so, I'm a 7.5! And they can keep spreading, especially at the front part, causing squeezing and numbness if the shoes do not allow for this change in size. These long, unstable feet have to carry a long, unstable body – little wonder that those with hEDS often end up in the podiatrist's chair...

## Basic Moves

Being able to sit and stand upright, and move easily about the world without having to think too much is something we tend to take for granted once we have progressed past crawling and toddling and broken into a run. Just consider, for a moment, getting from one side of the room to the other – navigating doors, tables, chairs and the cat – and you will realise just what a phenomenal job your body does every day. Held securely in just the right place with just the right amount of stretch and flex, your bones, muscles and all the trappings steer you nimbly around your surroundings. Solid, flat floors? Piece of cake. Soft, grassy parks? No worries – saunter along and enjoy the fresh air. A bit of a clamber over rocks to reach the top of that hill over there? A bit more to think about but...hurry up, slowcoach! The human with hEDS is having to think about each step. Her brain is working overtime trying to figure out how to keep everything going in the same direction as the tendons and ligaments stretch and those bones start slipping out of alignment. Muscles strain to keep the skeleton stable and, if she stops concentrating for a second, the whole lot might, quite literally, come tumbling down.

Simply standing still takes an effort on the part of the muscles to hold everything in place, and the strain of this can make the body ache. So those with hEDS will lean against walls, shift from one leg to another or just sit on the ground after quite brief periods of standing still in a queue or to have a chat in the street. When sitting down, the seemingly easy task of sitting up straight is tiring and so the body repeatedly slumps and, when that position starts to ache, the hEDSer will draw (or sometimes use their arms to push) themselves up to sitting up straight again before gradually rounding the back and shoulders once more as the effort to hold it together becomes too much to maintain. It is a mistake to think that those with hEDS simply need to 'strengthen those muscles' – those muscles are working out constantly and are often super-strong...it is the connections between them that are too lax, and pumping iron won't help that and might just cause an injury.

The overworking of one muscle group can cause an imbalance which can, in turn, lead to a joint popping out. You won't meet many hEDSers who can't regale you with a story of how they were busy following a rehabilitation programme to strengthen a muscle after an injury only to put out another joint and have to start all over again! Daily exercise is a cornerstone of protecting the hEDS body, but specialist physiotherapists working with clients with hEDS rarely encourage repetitive resistance training with weights and aim instead for a graduated strengthening programme.[5] Sure, lifting weights can help, but only if a very careful programme is followed to ensure that each and every muscle is powered up to pull just the right amount, in just the right direction, in perfect complement to the muscle on the other side of the joint. Overwork one muscle and expect a cascade of consequences.

People with hEDS often describe their journey through doors in their home as 'ping-ponging' – that doorway seems so impossibly narrow when you walk like a drunk on nothing more than a weak cup of tea. So we will bang against one side of the door frame and then, in an attempt to straighten up, we overcompensate and crash against the other side of the frame. Those of you old enough to remember the very first computer games will know now why we call it 'ping-ponging'. Personally I just wish my body made the same noise as that little white dot did when it hit the 'bat' on the opponent's side – that would provide endless amusement for all the family!

In order to gain stability, the hEDSer will unconsciously adopt various positions which might look odd but feel perfectly comfortable and normal to them. Sitting square on a kitchen chair, both feet on the ground might seem an obvious way to feel 'grounded' and stable for the average skeleton but is very wobbly when your hip bone just does not feel 'connected to your...thigh bone' and your thigh bone really does not feel 'connected to your...knee bone!' as the old song goes. So we might shift into a cock-eyed position, pop one foot up on the rung of another chair or turn one foot right onto its side on the floor to 'lock' it into a more stable position. As comfy as it feels at the time, as we will see in later chapters, there can be profound, lifelong implications for this repeated overstretching and abnormal alignment of limbs and joints. You can point it out to an hEDSer and they will probably have to look and check because they simply cannot feel that anything is odd. They lack...

## Proprioception

Now, as if the process of moving an overly loose body around wasn't hard enough, the sensors that tell us where we are in space are located in the muscles and joints. This ability to be able to know where our body is even with our eyes closed is called proprioception,[6] and proprioception in those with hEDS is, frankly, pants! To give you some idea of how well normal proprioception works, consider your life at university. In my experience, university beds are extra narrow (maybe to save on the cost of bigger sheets, maybe to give extra desk space and maybe to stop students ignoring their studies by laying in bed all day!). Now I suspect you enjoyed many a freshers' ball or nights down the student union bar sinking one too many cheap ciders and fell into bed much the worse for wear and, just possibly, in the company of another student also much the worse for wear: two overhydrated bodies in an undersized bed barely aware of their own names, let alone their nocturnal surroundings. And I bet you *still* didn't spend the night repeatedly falling out of bed. That is proprioception!

For those with hEDS the sense of where their limbs are in relation to their surroundings can be very altered and, although the exact reason for this is unclear, it has been suggested that affected joint and tendon receptors are the culprits.[7] This can make for a rather clumsy client. In addition, because humans can use visual clues to aid balance and proprioception, dark environments can prove particularly tricky to navigate for those with hEDS. The ears also play a part in balance and, as we will see in Chapter 5, these are also commonly affected with hEDS, adding to the overall mobility anarchy.

So the hEDS body has to work overtime to stay upright, struggles to work out where it is in space and, when it bangs into something, bruises more easily, and heals more slowly. It is difficult to describe the physical and mental toll this can have – day after day the simplest tasks require extra thought and vigilance and, despite our best efforts, we still end up crashing around getting bruised and injured. The brain, trying desperately to keep the body safe, works overtime and so the person with hEDS is often described as 'tired but wired' with that hypervigilant state leading to high anxiety levels (more about the mental health impact of hEDS in Chapter 8). As we have seen, many women with hEDS have spent a lifetime undiagnosed and so may well have grown up carrying various labels such as 'clumsy', 'neurotic', 'lazy' and 'fearful'. As a child I could never understand why I was simply unable to navigate my way like a young gazelle across the rocks on the beach to explore the rock pools. The rest of the family didn't even need to watch their feet it seemed, but my heart would pound with the thought of stepping down from one slippery rock to another. And then, at the edge of a deep rock pool I'd feel the need to hang on to someone else for fear I'd fall in. I have also laid down on my stomach and cried at the top of a hill, hanging on to the ground, unable to feel safe in the stiff wind. On the other hand, when I can't sleep at night, I often entertain myself by trying to guess where my arms and legs are – it is not uncommon for me to think my legs are lying parallel only to find, when I look, that they are crossed over each other and bent! Every cloud has a silver lining.

## Sprains and Strains

I once took my son to A&E with yet another sprained ankle ('He was playing with his father' being the common denominator) and he was greeted by name! I love a good Saturday evening in our local A&E – they have a TV and, one time, we watched the 1958 classic film *The Blob* when the hordes of injured rugby players and clubbers made for an overly long wait to be seen. Happy days!

The child with hEDS often grows up knowing exactly how to strap an ankle or wrist from an early age, so common are their sprains and strains. It isn't simply the joint instability causing the strain or sprain but the fact that the proprioception is altered – the perfect storm of a wobbly joint and the body's inability to judge how far out of alignment that joint is heading. Heavy falls can, of course, result in a broken bone but much more likely is that the loose ligaments will allow a bashed bone to slide around, hauling on the supportive tissues as it goes, causing soft tissue damage that might actually take a lot longer than a fracture to recover. Exercise is essential for the hEDS body to optimise strength and minimise pain and anxiety but you can see the daily dilemma...

Although hEDS itself doesn't appear to be associated with the onset of osteoarthritis, repeated injury to a joint has been shown to lead to an increased risk[8] which, in turn, can further limit mobility and increase anxiety and pain.

Although many with hEDS are looser than normal in all their joints, most have some joints that are significantly looser and more likely to sprain than others. One hEDSer might be very loose in the knees but a little less so in their ankles and vice versa, but there is often a knock-on effect with an injured ankle putting extra strain on the knee which subsequently starts playing up. It is tempting for the parents of a child with hEDS to want to protect them and 'wrap them up in cotton wool' but this approach can lead to a lifelong fear of exercise and potentially devastating deconditioning that can cause further instability and pain.

## Subluxations and Dislocations

As we have seen, the bones are held securely in alignment by a complex system of muscles, tendons, ligaments and connective tissue and, in those with hEDS, this system is under constant strain. The vastly over-worked muscles can start to work against each other and, given how stretchy the attached ligaments, tendons and other tissues are, it doesn't take much to pull a joint out of place. Clicking joints, subluxations (partial or incomplete dislocation) and full dislocations are much more common in the hEDS population than in the general population, with some 75 per cent of hEDSers reporting dislocations at some point in their life.[9] The most common joint affected appears to be the shoulder but, with instability throughout the entire musculoskeletal system, any joint can pop out. As we have already seen, the temporomandibular joint, being like the rest of the joints in the body rather loose, tends to clunk out of place rather easily, giving rise to TMJD with its implications for intubation and knock-on effects on the ears (see Chapter 5 for more about the ears, nose and throat (ENT)).

*I grew up thinking it was normal for your knee to slip out place when sitting for carpet time in school, so never made a fuss.*

Bex

Because the connective tissue is so lax and beyond tightening, once a joint has dislocated and the attached anchorings overstretched, repeat dislocations are a real risk, bringing accompanying pain and anxiety. It is understandable that this can lead to a fear of even the most gentle exercise, but the more deconditioned the hEDS body becomes, the more unstable and sore it is likely to be. Some hEDSers are prone to frequent, even daily, subluxations and dislocations, whilst for others it happens rarely. All of us experience frequent 'slides' as joints sublux, and bones ease out of place and then clunk back in without too much drama besides a yelp. I remember teaching a couple of my sons how to massage and wiggle their feet to help ease the little network of bones back into alignment when something feels 'all wrong'. Even for a minimally dislocating hEDSer a mis-timed cough can pop a rib out, making breathing very uncomfortable until it decides to get back home, kneecaps can take a wander if they're not concentrating coming downstairs, and an over-enthusiastic yawn can result in a painfully out of place jaw. Living with hEDS takes real courage at times, especially when we know that daily exercise is essential to reduce the likelihood of dislocations, whilst anticipating the exhaustion, injury and pain that we will experience along the reconditioning pathway.

*The pain started in my teenage years with lower back ache. Then I started getting ankle pain...then hip pain when walking. I kept going back to see my GP with various joint pains and it took years before a new GP looked over my notes and connected the dots, proposing EDS.*

Sophie

## Pelvic Girdle Pain

The pelvic girdle deserves a special mention for the obvious reason that this is a book for midwives and doulas. Sure, there are all the other joints in the body which are affected by hEDS but none are going to impact so much on the pregnancy and birth, and potentially, for many years after birth. The female pelvis is beautifully evolved to combine the need for safe pregnancy and childbirth alongside the ability to walk long distances at the same speed as their male counterparts (see Figure 2.1).[10] The main structure consists of two large hip bones which themselves each comprise three fused bones (the ilium, ischium and pubis). The two hip bones are held together at the back by the sacrum and coccyx (the sacral joints being one each side), and at the front the bones are kept in alignment by the cartilaginous symphysis pubis.[11] So, together, there are four joints within the bony pelvic girdle: the two sacroiliac joints where the hip bones meet the sacrum, the sacrococcygeal joint between the sacrum and the coccyx, and the symphysis pubis where the hip bones meet at the front. Outside of pregnancy the pelvis is really very stable and does its job of bearing and transferring the weight of the upper skeleton down through the lower part, providing attachment points for a variety of muscles and ligaments, and protecting the abdominal organs.

Pregnancy, of course, requires a slight slackening of the pelvic ligaments to allow just enough movement for descent, rotation and eventual birth of the baby whilst continuing to provide enough stability that the pregnant woman is able to maintain mobility reasonably comfortably. Needless to say, the overly lax ligaments that feature so large in the hEDS-affected pregnant woman can lead to destabilisation of the pelvic girdle and consequent pain and immobility. About 45 per cent of women are affected by pelvic girdle pain (PGP) in pregnancy[12] but that number rises to 88 per cent in those with hEDS,[13] often starting much earlier, and becoming more severe. Furthermore, whilst PGP generally resolves within a few months of giving birth, for those affected by hEDS the symptoms might continue for much longer, and sometimes for years,[14] as their ligaments continue to be too lax, whilst those in the general postnatal population gradually return to normal.

The pain of PGP can be all-encompassing and increases with walking, rolling over in bed, sleeping and load-bearing – just carrying a bag on the shoulder can be enough to cause pain. Destabilisation around the sacral joints can lead to irritation of the sciatic nerve, causing sciatica, whilst movement in the symphysis pubis can leave women feeling as if they have been kicked in the front by a horse.

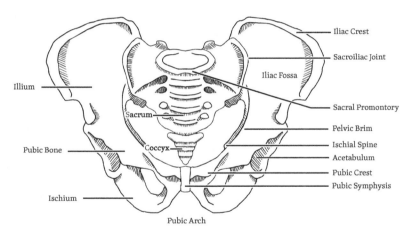

*Figure 2.1 The female pelvis*

Apart from the expected pain that is a feature of PGP, those with hEDS are likely to feel even more unstable than usual and will often describe feeling as if their whole pelvis is coming apart! As the woman walks she might feel the pelvic bones shifting quite alarmingly and, at the same time, be very aware of her femurs clunking in and out of their acetabula. Used as she is to being prone to stumbles and trips, this increased sense of instability can greatly increase the anxiety of the already anxious pregnant hEDSer. As we will see in Part II, the usual treatments such as using a pregnancy support belt might not prove so effective for the woman with hEDS and, with the propensity to heal more slowly, she might not be the ideal candidate for an elective caesarean section and so the hEDSer with PGP is likely to need a more personalised approach to care and rehabilitation.

## Breaks

As we have seen, the increased laxity of the supporting tissues can allow bones to shift about during a trip or fall, increasing the stretch on the already overstretched ligaments and tendons, and, in turn, leading to painful strains and sprains. Historically it has been assumed that bones get off scot-free in hEDS but we should remember that around 90 per cent of the bone matrix is made up of collagen and so we shouldn't be surprised if there is a degree of bone involvement in hEDS.[15]

Whilst bone mass density does not seem to be affected, there is growing evidence that the faulty collagen can cause a degree of increased bone fragility with a noted increased risk of vertebral fracture.[16] It is useful to remember that at the very far end of the faulty collagen continuum lies osteogenesis imperfecta (brittle bone disease) and there is some developing evidence of an overlap between some forms of EDS and this rare disease causing multiple fractures from birth in those affected, and that this overlap could represent a missing EDS subtype.[17] Rare though it is, when caring for a pregnant, labouring or newly birthed woman, it pays to be vigilant to the possibility of her baby being potentially more at risk of osteogenesis than a baby born to an hEDS-unaffected mother.

## Tendonitis and Bursitis

Tendonitis and bursitis are the painful inflammation and swelling of a tendon – the thick cord which tethers a muscle to a bone – or a bursa – the fluid-filled sac which acts as a cushion between bones and the tendons or muscles surrounding the bone. Both conditions are more common in those with hEDS.[18] Tendonitis and bursitis are generally caused by repetitive overuse of a joint (repetitive strain injury, or RSI) or by a sudden, sharp movement causing irritation and minor injury to the tissues. The person with hEDS, as we have seen, is often blissfully unaware of where her limbs are in relation to where they should, more correctly, lie. Consider an hEDSer spending an evening in front of the TV enjoying a spot of knitting. There is the repetitive action but, in addition, as she knits, her elbows, wrists and fingers will all be stretching beyond where nature intended, over and over and over. It feels quite OK at the time – remember that there is a loss of proprioception and so the knitter has no idea that her joints are doing anything strange or exaggerated – but the next day...

If you ask the hEDSer with a splinted wrist what they've done, you might well get a shrug and 'I really have no idea'!

## Plantar Fasciitis and Morton's Neuroma

Having travelled right down the body, considering each part of the musculoskeletal system and how the lack of stability in both the joints and the tissues can give rise to a multitude of conditions, with no part of the body untouched, it seems right and proper to end at the foot. We have seen how the hEDS feet might be long and thin and unusually flat, and on the ends of overly flexible ankles which have a tendency to turn and wrench at the slightest provocation. Over the years, those stretchy, bendy feet can hurt...really hurt. Those with hEDS can suffer considerably more than the average population with their feet[19] and require ongoing and increasing support as they reach adulthood. Most notable of those painful conditions are plantar fasciitis and Morton's neuroma.

The first of these, plantar fasciitis,[20] is a condition where the fibrous ligament connecting the heel to the front of, and supporting the arch of, the foot becomes inflamed – more likely with the repeated overstretch- ing caused by the flattened hEDS foot arch. Once warmed up with a little gentle walking, the plantar fascia eases up and the pain lessens, but those first few minutes of the day or after a period of hiking, oh my word – putting one foot after another can feel like walking on hot coals. This condition can be exacerbated by increased weight so pregnancy can be particularly grim and plantar fasciitis is notoriously resistant to treatment. It often spontaneously disappears but not until after a few miserable years of hopping around howling in the mornings.

Morton's neuroma is a benign thickening of the tissue that sur- rounds the digital nerve leading to the toes.[21] It commonly affects the area between the third and fourth toes causing pain and a sensation of walking 'on a marble'. As it worsens, walking can become impossible due to the pain, even with good shoes and orthotic insoles; if that fails to give lasting relief, steroid injections followed by surgery can sometimes be the only answers to get a sufferer mobile again. As with plantar fasciitis, the flat, hypermobile feet, struggling to support an overly flexible hEDS body, cause undue strain on more fragile, slow to heal tissues, leaving inflammation, pain and the potentially long-term damage of a Morton's neuroma.

So from the top of the church roof palate down to the ingrown toenails and Morton's neuroma, the hEDS musculoskeletal system can seem like one huge collection of problems. I often think of hEDS as a 'bucket syndrome'; those with hEDS, trying to recover from one injury whist busy picking up another, head full of various treatment plans they are supposed to be following, sometimes stare down into their overflowing bucket and wonder where to start.

CHAPTER 3

# The Cardiovascular System

## Introduction

The cardiovascular system is the body's transport system for blood. The heart as the key organ of the system is the fist-sized muscle which contracts rhythmically and autonomously ensuring a continuous circulation of blood around the body via an extensive network of blood vessels and capillaries running throughout the body.[1] The flow direction of blood around the heart and body is controlled by valves – four within the heart itself and an additional variable number in the veins,[2] whilst blood pressure is regulated by a combination of the strength of the heart muscle, vascular tone and health, and hormonal activity.

When we start to focus on the circulation of the blood around the body, it is easy to forget the other essential part of the system – the lungs. We tend to think of the lungs as the main organ of the respiratory system – which of course they are – but they also form part of the circulatory system, taking the role of oxygenating the blood before it zips around the body to deliver its package to every single cell, and without which they would quickly die.

The heart and lungs work seamlessly together, driven through a series of nervous and chemical interactions that fall completely outside our conscious control via the autonomic nervous system. Bundles of nerves, and sensitive chemical receptors in and around the brain, heart and lungs monitor the pH of the blood for levels of carbon dioxide and oxygen, adjusting the rate and strength of the heartbeat and the rate and depth of breathing accordingly, thereby maintaining a steady state – homeostasis.[3]

From the moment the embryonic heart makes its first tiny beat until the end of life, the heart and lungs work in tandem to ensure a smooth running of our body no matter what we are putting it through. Whether we are running for a bus or enjoying a leisurely read over a cuppa, concentrating furiously on the trickiest work challenge or knocking out the zeds at 2 a.m., our heart, lungs and vascular system ensure the correct heart and respiration rate to keep us, quite literally, ticking over.

The ubiquity of collagen throughout the body means that the entire circulatory system, including the lungs, can be affected in hEDS. As you will see in Chapter 8 on the autonomic nervous system, even the ability to breathe without thinking can be somewhat out of kilter, but the focus of the present chapter is on the effects of those stretchy tissues on the secure working of blood circulation.

*My resting heart rate is high, blood pressure is low and core temperature is low. This has always baffled medical professionals whose knowledge on EDS is limited.*

Lottie

At this point it is sensible to consider why it is vital that EDS is not seen as one single syndrome but, as we explored in Chapter 1, a group of 13 subtypes, and that each client with EDS is treated according to their individual subtype. Although all subtypes share the same basic fault in collagen, making it more fragile and stretchy than it should be, the degree and way that is expressed throughout the various organs and systems of the body varies. So whilst those with hEDS might have very thin and unusual scarring, it is those with the classic subtype (cEDS) who are often so significantly scarred that they can have skin discolouration, particularly on their shins and elbows. Those with hEDS may experience issues with their teeth, but it is the periodontal subtype (pEDS) which hones in on teeth and gums with profound impacts on dentition from an early age. Likewise, whilst those with hEDS may well have various issues with their heart, lungs and vascular system, it is vascular EDS (vEDS) where there is such significant impact that the condition generally limits life expectancy, with the median age of death at just 48 years from aortic or organ rupture.[4]

When a woman presents for pregnancy booking and declares that

STRETCHED TO THE LIMITS

she has a diagnosis of hEDS, many practitioners only hear the EDS part. Some will not have the faintest clue what EDS is and head off to do a spot of googling and quite often hit on classic EDS first, whilst others will have come across it before but maybe a different subtype and simply conflate one with the other. A client with cEDS is a candidate for obstetric care whilst one with hEDS without any other conditions really might do better with low-tech midwife care and, if the last client with EDS an obstetrician saw had the vascular subtype then the simple hEDS client can quickly find herself on entirely the wrong care pathway through a process of medical Chinese whispers. I have lost count of the number of times I have known a client with hEDS be told she was at higher risk of cervical incompetence or uterine rupture when neither of these things are true. The woman with hEDS has high enough anxiety as it is without being scared half to death by well-meaning but uninformed health care professionals. The situation is not made any easier by the general confusion over where the two most common subtypes (hEDS and cEDS) converge and diverge, meaning that most hEDS women I've had contact with seem to end up being treated as if they have cEDS.

So, back to the circulation and lungs...

## Heart

As we have seen, the heart is a powerful muscle, beautifully evolved to keep blood pumping around the one way-system of arteries, veins and capillaries and with a series of valves to ensure there is no backwash along the route. Although the evidence is mixed, it appears that the incidence of both valvular incompetence and conductivity irregularities is increased in those with hEDS.[5] This is not surprising given the presence of collagen in the heart valves. Most hEDSers are very familiar with palpitations and 'skipped beats' and may well have experienced them regularly since early childhood. If one or other parent was affected then they might have been brought up to think it was perfectly normal. Certainly I was told not to worry about those 'flip-flops' in my chest as a young child because 'they're normal – everyone gets them!' Alongside those ectopic beats can come a sudden lack of a beat or two, or a sudden short burst of tachycardia – enough to cause a weird need to 'cough it away' before a swimmy dizziness grips. It is arguable that this 'normalising' approach might help children growing up with hEDS, enabling them to take part in activities without the anxiety that the occasionally irregular tick of their heart spells trouble. The parent who has not themselves experienced an hEDS heart rate as a youngster might be inclined to panic when faced with their child's questions about palpitations and pathologise them, raising their anxiety levels and limiting their exercise which can, paradoxically, worsen hEDS symptoms.

The majority of heart rate irregularities in hEDS are caused by the impact of the condition on the autonomic nervous system affecting conductivity, and we look at the ANS in detail in Chapter 8. There may be an associated mitral valve regurgitation caused by increased stretchiness of the tissues,[6] but it is likely to be mild and of little consequence. However, due to the increased workload on the heart posed by pregnancy and labour, it is worth keeping in mind the possibility of valve involvement.

*I'm a good singer and swimmer and can control my lungs really well for that, but cannot run or exercise and breathe! I was diagnosed with inappropriate sinus tachycardia which the cardiologist explained means my heart does what it wants when it wants and doesn't respond in a 'normal' way to my body's nervous system.*

Nicole

## Veins, Arteries and Capillaries

The serious impact of EDS on blood vessels is seen in the rarer subtypes of EDS, such as the vascular type vEDS. For the hEDS community the effects are life-affecting and not life-threatening.

The majority of impact of hEDS on the circulatory system is in the outer reaches – the veins, arteries and capillaries – and, although not completely understood (due in part to the lack of rigorous study), the most likely explanation is the obvious one: soft vessel walls allowing pooling of blood to take place.[7] For all humans, remaining conscious whilst upright requires the blood vessels around the body to allow and aid good blood flow back to the lungs for oxygenation and the heart

STRETCHED TO THE LIMITS

for pumping back round again. When this system breaks down, even a little, symptoms can emerge.

So the client with hEDS, possessing soft-walled blood vessels, is very much more prone to pooling of the blood and this is not helped by the increased laxity in the vein valves and the lack of firm structure in the surrounding connective tissue – those usual back-up systems ensuring the blood pressure and flow is tickety-boo. Those with hEDS commonly live with ongoing daily symptoms of low blood pressure even when not standing for long periods. Most hEDSers complain of daily brain fog[8] and poor memory as well as significant 'head rush' with quite moderate changes of position or when stepping out of a hot atmosphere into a cooler one. Chest pains, visual disturbances (a kind of hazy and short-term 'greying-out'), shakiness, intolerance to exercise and then feeling worse after exercise, feeling worse after a big meal, ankle oedema after standing for short periods of time, cold hands and feet, and just ('just!') general tiredness.[9] Notably, we also make notoriously cheap drunks as, drug intolerance aside (more of that in the next chapter), whilst a high intake of alcohol can increase blood pressure, to get there you have to start with the one or two drinks which can actually lower blood pressure a wee bit[10] and many of us with hEDS react so much that we never get any further – take us out for a night and save yourself some money! A few years ago I bought my husband a birthday treat of a day at a real ale festival. I asked on the way in if they did thirds of a pint and, happy days, they did. So I made sure to eat before each third of a pint and to sip the amber nectar as if it were an expensive whiskey and managed a whole pint over the space of about seven hours. I felt so rough that I had to sleep it off all evening!

Now, all the above symptoms are par for the course in a day for someone with poorly regulated blood pressure. Once a bit of prolonged standing is introduced things can get tricky – intolerance to standing, apparent anyway in hEDSers due to those lax joints and shoddy proprioception, is compounded by the bigger, more sustained drop in blood pressure leading to a tendency to light headedness (pre-syncope) and even fainting (syncope). The efforts of the heart to rectify matters can sometimes lead to a rather over-enthusiastic rise in heart rate leading to a postural orthostatic tachycardic episode.[11] More about postural orthostatic tachycardia syndrome (POTS) in Chapter 8 when we explore the autonomic nervous system but, put simply, the person stands up, blood pressure drops and the heart rate increases and, although a rise in heart rate is a normal bodily response to a drop in blood pressure, in hEDS it can all get exaggerated, kicking in too easily and too thoroughly. Mild POTS symptoms can be felt at any time on a bad EDS day (you will hear those with hEDS say they feel 'a bit POTSy today'), whilst a significant attack of POTS can strike when stood for a period of time or when suddenly going from sitting to standing.

Anything that has a tendency to lower blood pressure is likely to have a greater impact on those with hEDS and really exacerbate POTS: sleep, heat, certain medications and alcohol, eating a big meal, following a low-salt diet, dehydration, standing and pregnancy... The woman with hEDS chugging down her own body weight in sports drinks and crisps isn't in need of a lecture on healthy eating – she is simply trying to keep herself from passing out!

Paradoxically, whilst low blood pressure can cause daytime tiredness and brain fog, it can also cause poor sleep at night. Blood pressure drops overnight in any case by around 10–20 per cent and then rises as morning approaches. Excessive nocturnal hypotension can cause a reactive picture, robbing the sufferer of much-needed rest – the drop in blood pressure can cause some deoxygenating and hypoglycaemia of the brain and so the body kicks awake to push the blood pressure back up, normal service is resumed, sleep ensues and the cycle rinses and repeats.[12] In addition, that low blood pressure can also cause a tripping-in of a tachycardia and a feeling of being 'jump-started' awake. 'Tired but wired' can become the natural lived experience of the client with hEDS.

The softness of the veins and surrounding supportive tissues can cause issues other than low blood pressure. Veins have a tendency to collapse more easily, making phlebotomy more of a trial for all involved – a brachial vein can look amazingly tempting bulging away under the thin and stretchy skin, but the second a firm metal needle touches it, it comes over all shy and retiring, refusing all attempt to coax it back to give up its bounty. There will sometimes be just one reliable bleeder which doesn't collapse and it is easy to spot due to the scarring from overuse!

*I become quite the challenge for phlebotomists – the needle goes in and 'Uh, oh!', the vein has shifted.*

Bekah

Varicosities are more common (a history of varicose veins forms part of the Beighton criteria[13]) – every size available from large varicose veins right down to tiny spider veins in the legs, anal varicosities in the form of internal and external haemorrhoids and, during pregnancy, vulval varicosities can be more of a likelihood. The thinness and easy compression of the covering skin can make damage to smaller, more fragile veins easier so that even picking up a pen a little too firmly, or holding a can opener handle over a small vein might cause a little venule (size-wise somewhere between a vein and a capillary) in a finger to break and bleed under the surface. They come up fast and hurt like heck and sometimes they clot, sclerose and then hang around for months or years, reminding you to let someone else open the can of beans next time.

*I have a few abdominal vascular compressions that restrict my ability to eat comfortably and maintain a healthy body weight.*

Claire

A history of recurrent nosebleeds is another common feature.[14] There is no history of just a bang to the nose or a good old pick causing the bleed – the nose simply starts bleeding and, once stopped, it tends to be easier to re-start. Once out of childhood, heavy periods can be more common.[15] And yet blood tests will show that platelet levels and the clotting profile is completely normal.

From the large pumping sergeant of the heart down to the tiniest foot soldier, the capillary system is the much-forgotten jewel in the circulatory crown. Capillaries are gloriously brilliant tiny blood vessels comprising around 10 billion in number which join the arteries and veins together whilst being thin-walled enough to allow oxygen and nutrients to pass to organs, tissues and cells and transport carbon dioxide and waste away from them. They are so thin that blood cells have to travel in single file along them. Given that collagen is an important component of capillary structure, it will come as no surprise that they break more easily in someone with EDS.[16] Bruising, as we saw in Chapter 1, is a feature of all EDS subtypes including hEDS, although the severity varies between the subtypes, and, as you know, women tend to bruise more easily than men. Expect your hEDS client to tell you that she is 'a bit of a bruiser'. The thinness of the skin will also allow the bruise to show more and for longer and, unprotected as it is by a stronger layer of skin, it might well be pretty tender.

Capillary fragility can also give rise to the easy formation of petechiae which can be alarming when the trauma causing the rash has been so slight. I have a fabulous photo of my thighs the morning after a scout camp fire when I'd been leading a yodelling, thigh-slapping song. Despite wearing good jeans my thighs were absolutely black and blue with a petechial rash clearly showing my hand prints. But a random bit of thigh-slapping isn't needed to kick up a petechial rash – just scratching or carrying a shopping bag over the forearms will do it, and yet platelets and clotting factors are normal in the hEDS client.

*When I cough hard or retch all the capillaries around my eyes burst, leaving little red dots that last a few days.*

Anna

Alongside easier bleeding and bruising, slower wound healing is a feature across the whole EDS family, with the rarer subtypes being far more badly affected.[17] The client with cEDS is likely to have more issues with slow and abnormal wound healing but again, with your hEDS client, although less likely to be as affected in terms of wound healing as the client with cEDS, she is still more likely to have slower healing than the general population and this should be considered during care-planning. It cannot be stressed strongly enough that there is *not* a problem with clotting – platelets are as likely to be normal in someone with hEDS as in someone without it – it is the fragility of the skin, vessels and capillaries that is the problem.

## Lungs

Although part of the same system, and often affected in hEDS, we will look at the trachea, larynx and pharynx in Chapter 5 on the ears, nose and throat.

The two lungs sit above the diaphragm, placed either side of the heart. They are protected by the rib cage and each is located within its own fluid-filled and lubricating pleural cavity.[18] The function of the lungs is to oxygenate the blood and, in turn, every cell in the body. As with heartbeat, breathing is under the control of the autonomic nervous system. However, unlike the heart, as we all know, it is possible to take control of the breathing. The most serious effects on the lungs from EDS are seen in those with the vascular type who are at risk of spontaneous pneumothorax and haemothorax, whilst for those with hEDS the main respiratory symptoms are exertional dyspnoea, sleep apnoea, voice changes and asthma.[19]

The super-stretchy lung tissues alongside flexible vocal cords can lend themselves to a genuine plus of hEDS, namely that the community is renowned for producing good singers! The stretchy lungs can significantly increase the lung capacity – I am often struck by how many in the hEDS community say they breathe much more slowly than their partners – but the soft nature of the tissues means that both the upper and lower airways are more likely to collapse on expiration.[20] The fragile tissues are more prone to irritation and tiredness so laryngitis, hoarseness (with or without infection), coughing and hay fever are also common, especially as those with hEDS are more likely to be atopic (atopy being that inherited family of asthma, eczema, hay fever and migraine). The cause of hEDS cough and hoarseness can be a little tricky to pin down due to the prevalence of gastro-oesophageal reflux in this population but digging down into the increased number of asthmatics in the hEDS population throws up the notion that, rather than the asthma being of the usual pathology, the cause might more likely be down to the altered structure of the lung collagen itself.[21]

As outlined in Chapter 2, the musculoskeletal system, working overtime to stay in alignment and upright, can tire and ache more than general and so rib and back pain are extremely common in those with hEDS. When sitting up straight requires constant effort and vigilance, it is easy to slump and the altered proprioception means that there isn't always an awareness that the body has crumpled, leading to ongoing shallow breathing when sat down or resting which does nothing to improve the brain fog.

All of this is apparent in the hEDS client who is *not* pregnant. Little wonder then that having another human share the internal body space and pushing upwards on the lungs and heart, and putting an extra burden on the circulation, can spell trouble...

## CHAPTER 4

# The Gastrointestinal System

## Introduction

The human gastrointestinal (GI) tract starts at the mouth and finishes at the anus and comprises everything in between and the associated salivary and gastric glands.[1] The entire gastric tract from end to end is around nine metres long when at rest, which, in reality, it never is! Constantly in a state of waving muscular contractions, moving food and fluids along its length, extracting everything the body needs to survive and thrive, the GI tract is a veritable workhorse of a system.

The major component of the intestines, giving it its lovely stretchy quality, is collagen.[2] Nine metres of collagen-rich human tissue, residing in a human with a genetic condition affecting collagen synthesis and repair...what could possibly go wrong? Given the size and nature of the GI tract, it is not really surprising that a significant proportion of those with hEDS experience problems and that these span a range of issues.

Not only is collagen an essential component of the intestines themselves, it also surrounds the nerves serving them. The faulty nature of this nerve-enveloping collagen seems to cause those with hEDS to be more sensitive to the workings of the gut.[3] This means that not only can the gut be more functionally affected but that the owner of the gut actually can feel the gut functioning (well or otherwise) more acutely than the average person, so that they are symptomatic without having any GI pathology. As if that wasn't enough, as we will see in Chapter 8 on the autonomic nervous system, dysregulation of central nervous system processing can cause the nerves serving the GI system to get their wires crossed so that it doesn't know if it is coming or going!

*Sometimes, I'll get an excruciating pain in my guts just before I need to poop, as if things are shifting around but in such a painful way.*

Sophie P

Disorders of the GI system are rife in the hEDS community with many experiencing an array of problems. So, although we will look one at a time at the most common issues, your client might well be suffering from any combination of them and might have been given a 'bucket' diagnosis of functional gastrointestinal disorder.[4]

## Hiatus Hernia

Once the food has made it out of the mouth into the oesophagus, the first hurdle to get past is the diaphragm and, needless to say, the softer collagen increases the likelihood of hiatus hernia in those with hEDS[5] with its delights of acid reflux and indigestion. Even in the absence of a hernia, the increased sensitivity of the GI tract can cause discomfort around eating. It can feel as if food simply isn't going down – sometimes it isn't but on other occasions, the oesophagus is simply feeling too much. The softer tissues both making up and surrounding the oesophagus and rest of the gastrointestinal tract can lead to little kinks along the way and this feels very obvious when it is the oesophagus that is momentarily affected.

*It's sometimes really hard to swallow my food too, as the muscles in my oesophagus become all confused and don't work together properly?*

Joey

Of course, there are plenty of lifestyle changes that can be made to ease the symptoms of reflux and hiatus hernia (eating little and often, not eating last thing at night, losing weight, avoiding trigger foods and taking medications) and I haven't come across many in the hEDS community who have not adjusted their dietary habits numerous times in an effort to reduce symptoms.

## Abnormal Gastric Emptying (Dysmotility)

If you imagine the stomach and intestines and the way the whole system works to move food through from top to bottom (quite literally), it is easy to see how things can get snarled up when hEDS is at play. The combination of stretchy tissues alongside faulty nerve messaging can create a myriad of often paradoxical symptoms. The stomach can be unusually slow to empty into the intestines, giving a sense of feeling too full after meals and feeling nauseous and uncomfortable with bloating and heartburn.[6] Some suffer with vomiting after big meals as the stomach simply won't empty its load fast enough and, although rare and the link is difficult to prove, some hEDSers suffer with gastroparesis, requiring more significant intervention than simple medications and lifestyle changes.

For some hEDSers there is an opposite effect and the stomach empties too fast, which can trigger POTS symptoms of sweating, shaking, rapid heart rate and feeling faint after eating a meal.[7] For others there is a very much more mixed picture with some slow days and some rapid days and some 'normal' days. Often a lot of energy goes into trying to disentangle what causes which reaction without ever finding out for sure because the system is simply out of whack. Of course, stress can affect the working of the guts so this constant search for strategies and solutions to the daily intestinal complaining only adds to the misery, but not thinking about it doesn't change the genetics and so hEDSers can find themselves in a double-bind.

## Constipation

The stretchy and over-sensitive intestines can allow food to hang around for longer than ideal, fluid gets re-absorbed and constipation results. This process (or lack of it) is made worse by the effects of hEDS on the serving nerves and, as you'd expect in a population who experience almost daily pain, the use of opiates. Sure, you can eat your own body weight in fibre or take 'bulk-forming' medications but that isn't a huge help if the bowel simply won't do its thing and get stuff moving. Constipation affects somewhere around 15–20 per cent of the general population and possibly around 35 per cent in the hEDS population, so this is a considerable problem within that community.[8] It cannot be stressed enough that this is not your average sort of constipation caused by poor diet, lack of adequate hydration and a sedentary lifestyle. All those things might be true for someone with hEDS but, even when you rectify all those with a treatment plan, you are still left with a genetic glitch that stops the system working as smoothly as it should.

*I have to remind myself that everything stretches, including my insides: if my guts stretch then they take longer to feel full, if they take longer to feel full then my body takes longer to realise I need to empty them out. This all results in chronic constipation.*

Naomi

## Irritable Bowel Syndrome

Irritable bowel syndrome (IBS) describes a condition whereby the sufferer experiences a combination of bloating, gas, intermittent bouts of cramps, constipation, diarrhoea or both. There may be painful constipation in the morning, bouts of diarrhoea in the evening and cramps in between. Others with IBS mainly suffer with constipation and are rarely troubled by diarrhoea, or vice versa. Diagnosed in around 11–15 per cent of the population, the condition is more common in women and very common in those with hEDS (with over 50% possibly affected).[9] The cause of IBS is a little unclear but there does seem to be a nervous connection and it is no accident, I guess, that this condition used to be called 'spastic colon' or 'nervous colon'. So with the hypersensitivity of the bowel in hEDS it might be that we really are very much more aware of the normal churning of our guts alongside the problems of abnormal motility. One of the more popular approaches to IBS currently is the adoption of the FODMAP diet. This is always known by its acronym for obvious reasons once you realise just what it entails – following a short-term diet low in fermentable oligosaccharides, disaccharides, monosaccharides and polyols. The idea is to reduce the workload on the gut by cutting down on foods that are harder to break down such as some fruits, dairy and wheat products. It is very specific and there are plenty of downloadable diet sheets to follow. It requires quite a degree of commitment but does seem to reward some IBS patients with relief from symptoms,[10] so you might well come across its use in your practice with hEDS clients. In order to 'switch off' the brain from noticing the sensations of the bowel action, and to ease some of the understandable anxiety of having IBS, cognitive behavioural therapy (CBT) is also now recommended.[11]

## Odd Gut Twists

One of the very odd side effects of having a stretchy bowel is that, sometimes, something as simple as a cough or sneeze can cause a sudden twisting in the bowel. It doesn't hurt exactly and it isn't like a muscle twitch or fasciculation, but it does make you grab your belly and shout a bit – such a strange feeling which hangs around for maybe half a minute, and then the intestine seems to unravel itself again and…it's gone! I hadn't realised it was 'a thing' until I sneezed during a physio appointment, doubled over and then, when asked if I was OK, said, 'You know when you sneeze and a bit of intestines gets in a twist for a little while?' Happily my physio is an hEDS specialist and was able to reassure me that, no, it wasn't a regular thing and, yes, it happens to the stretchy, nervous hEDS guts.

## Visceroptosis

It never ceases to amaze me how those metres of intestines manage to stay up, in place, defeating gravity and trampolines, rather than sinking unhappily to the pit of the abdomen to sulk their days away. The hero of the hour, quite literally doing all the heavy lifting of the guts, is the peritoneum, a large, complexly folded serous membrane which wraps around the stomach, intestines and other abdominal organs and holds them in place.[12] As well as its role as supporter in chief, this amazing organ also acts as a conduit for vessels, nerves and lymphatics, and has a part to play in immunity. The peritoneum consists of a layer of mesothelium supported by a thin layer of connective tissue and is divided into various parts, each with fabulous names – my all-time favourite being the one which sounds like a famous wrestler, The Greater Omentum!

The sheer range of gastrointestinal symptoms experienced by those with hEDS is understandable when you consider the size of the organs involved and the volume of connective tissue inherent in their make-up, and, although the studied numbers appear to be small, it is worth wondering if, at least for some affected individuals, looser peritoneal support due to more fragile and stretchy collagen within the peritoneum might exacerbate the situation still further by allowing the intestines to sag out of their normal position (visceroptosis).[13] There is still so much to know about EDS which might throw light on and answer some of the many questions we have about the experience of living in our bodies.

## Prolapse

That wholesale lack of support within the very tissues that are supposed to give it means that those with any connective tissue condition, including hEDS, are at increased risk of prolapse.[14] As with other challenges faced by the whole EDS community, those with the hypermobile type are generally less severely affected than those with the rarer subtypes, but even a mild prolapse can be miserable, especially in pregnancy and birth, and so should not be overlooked. When prolapse affects the bowels, the unlucky owner might find themselves afflicted by a rectocele or rectal prolapse. With a rectocele, the weakness is in the posterior wall of the vagina, allowing the rectum to sag and bulge into the vagina. With a rectal prolapse by contrast, the weakness is in the rectal muscles, allowing the rectum to prolapse down into or out of the anus itself. Both conditions cause rectal pressure and discomfort and problems with opening the bowels, and a rectocele can also cause pain during sex. As with many of the other challenges faced by those with hEDS, the usual treatments of avoiding constipation, strengthening the pelvic floor and managing weight might need much longer to work and, as there is the constant battle against genetically messed-up collagen, be less effective.

## Mast Cell Activation Disorder

Although caused by a faulty reaction of the immune system rather than an inherent problem with the intestines themselves, because of the impact on the guts, and of the close association between gastrointestinal health and the secure working of the immune system,[15] we will look at food allergies (and intolerances) here and, in particular, the role played by mast cell activation disorder (MCAD).

Along with their increased risk of atopy, those with hEDS have a significantly increased risk of food and drug allergies and intolerances and there is also some evidence of an increased risk of coeliac disease.[16] Food intolerances occur when the gut has trouble digesting a certain food. Although miserable, they are not life-threatening and can come and go over time. Causing bloating, discomfort and gas, common villains of the gut peace are wheat and dairy, although pretty much any food, or chemical in food, can upset the sensitive gut. It is notoriously difficult to work out which food is causing the problem – most meals are made up of so many different ingredients after all – and it is all too easy, given the sporadic nature of symptoms, to see a causative relationship between a food substance and symptoms when, in fact, it is just smoke and mirrors. With hEDS and the incidence for some of POTS following meals, sorting out the wheat from the chaff can be even trickier.

Allergies arise as a result of an exaggerated immune response to a normally harmless substance. Whereas an intolerance can undoubtably be life-affecting, an allergy can prove to be life-threatening. Generally a substantial amount of a food is needed to trigger an intolerance response whilst an allergic response can be triggered by the very tiniest particle of the offending allergen. As with an intolerance, almost any food substance can cause allergy, but common offenders are nuts, eggs, fish and milk. In recent years there has been a growing interest and practice in exposure therapy whereby a body's tolerance to an allergen is increased by giving regular, tiny amounts of it in a controlled manner.[17] Rather than curing or reversing the allergy, this treatment simply decreases the likelihood of a life-threatening reaction should an unexpected exposure occur. In the meantime, careful avoidance of the trigger and carrying antihistamines and adrenaline is the daily management approach of those with an allergy or at risk of anaphylaxis.

So where do mast cells fit into this picture? Produced in the bone marrow, mast cells live in various areas of the body including the gut. They form part of the immune system and release histamine and other chemicals into the blood when they detect the presence of an allergen. The release of histamine in response to pollen causes those familiar symptoms of sneezing, watery eyes, runny nose…basically anything to help us wash out the allergen.[18] Within the gut, in response to a food allergen, they can cause cramps, bloating and diarrhoea – again, in the body's attempt to get rid of the problem food. But mast cells can go into overdrive, releasing large volumes of histamine and causing the recognisable symptoms of an allergic response – flushing, swelling of the tissues, difficulty breathing and shock.

When my boys were young they used to love a good water fight. Armed with washing-up liquid bottles and water pistols they'd hare about the garden having the time of their life. Naturally their dad couldn't feel left out, so before long the hose would be brought out and the nonsense would increase. Then, on one memorable day, in a ridiculous fit of parental over-enthusiasm, my bloke grabbed the entire paddling pool which had been providing some cool relief for us all, and, adrenaline coursing through his veins, managed to upend the entire contents in one fell swoop over the boys! I watched, a mixture of delight and horror as all four children were swept across the lawn on a tsunami of their father's making...that kind of looks like my image of mast cell overdrive!

Mast cell activation disorder (MCAD) refers to an increase in mast cells, an increase in the activity of mast cells, or both. There is growing interest in the association between MCAD and connective tissue disorders, particularly hEDS.[19] Primarily, when affected, the hEDS population has overactive rather than over-numerous mast cells and impacted individuals can experience allergy-type responses quite randomly. Sometimes it is impossible to find a trigger and sometimes a trigger is suspected which was not a trigger a month ago. Something as simple as walking into a room where someone is wearing perfume might spell trouble for someone with MCAD. For some the symptoms are of daily, itchy rashes and a runny nose along with abdominal discomfort. Others may have wheezing and swelling and even full-blown anaphylaxis. Those hEDSers with POTS are the most likely in the EDS population to be affected by MCAD, but even those without POTS can be afflicted by it. There is no cure, and treatment with antihistamines, a low-histamine diet and other medications tends to bring only patchy relief.

## Local Anaesthetics

For reasons which are not yet known, somewhere between 60 and 80 per cent of people with hEDS have an insufficient effect from local anaesthetic.[20] They need a lot more than the general public to have sufficient effect and the anaesthesia tends to wear off more quickly. This obviously has implications for a range of medical and dental situations, none more so than in obstetrics and midwifery.

## Nutritional Deficiencies

You can see that those with hEDS can have a range of gut issues and, whilst some only suffer from one complaint, many more will experience plenty and will have spent years trying to improve their symptoms. With intestines that play up at the slightest provocation and their owner jumping through various dietary and pharmaceutical hoops in an attempt to find relief, it is tricky to know whether it is the erratic functioning of the intestines themselves, a diet that is in a perpetual state of analysis and adjustment, or the necking of a cocktail of meds that causes so many hEDSers to fret about the possibility of nutritional deficiencies, but I suspect the food supplement market loves us! Evidence is very hard to come by of any link between hEDS and nutritional deficiencies in the absence of dietary restrictions or the long-term use of specific medications, and I suspect that any particular vitamin or mineral deficiency is more as a result of a restrictive diet than just a natural by-product of faulty collagen.[21] But, in any case, safe to say that your hEDS client may well present rattling from her ingested collection of multivits and supplements!

From mouth to backside the hEDS gut can be a misery and, as that pregnancy test turns positive, it might well be about to get a whole lot worse...

CHAPTER 5

# Ears, Nose and Throat

## Introduction

It is so easy to get sidelined into the joint flexibility stuff when studying hEDS. After all, that is what is in the 'shop window' for all to see and, sure, the pain from repeatedly overstretched joints and dislocations can be exhausting to say the least. But, as you will be starting to gather now, the hidden stuff, the 'under the bonnet' stuff, can, at times, feel overwhelming yet often gets missed as part of the whole picture. So hEDSers end up going from pillar to post with an array of miserable symptoms throughout their body and seeing specialists from a huge spectrum of medical disciplines and the dots too often simply don't get joined up.

So it is when it comes to the area of ears, nose and throat (ENT). The EDS collagen-affecting impacts on the sound working of the ears, nose and throat are now becoming an area of interest and making it into the medical literature but, in my work, I am still concerned that so many hEDSers I speak to struggle with a variety of ENT issues without anyone having connected them to their diagnosis of hEDS.

## Ears

The process of hearing is utterly fascinating. Just thinking about how sound waves reach our ears, get converted into electrical signals and then get converted back into recognisable sounds is simply mind-boggling and quite delightful.[1] Even understanding how it happens, it makes me smile every time I think about it. And, understanding those marvellous intricacies can really help us get our heads around what is happening when hEDS puts obstacles in the way.

The process of hearing starts with the actual ear itself gathering and focusing the sound waves into the ear canal and along to the eardrum.

The eardrum vibrates just the right amount and passes those minute movements along the chain to the other side of the drum where we find the middle ear.

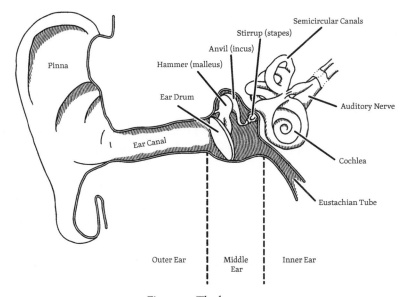

*Figure 5.1 The human ear*

This area contains the smallest bones in the body – the malleus, incus and stapes (great names for celebrity triplets, don't you think?) – with the malleus being in contact with the eardrum and then the other two being in close alignment, finishing with the stapes sitting in the connecting tissue between the middle and inner ear. The tiny ossicles themselves are held within the connective tissue of the middle ear, which allows just enough movement to transfer the vibrations created by the sound waves to the inner ear accurately.

The inner ear contains the fluid-filled organ of both hearing and balance – the cochlea. The vibrations from the stapes make the fluid inside the cochlea move, which, in turn, makes tiny little hairs inside the cochlea move. These tiniest of hair movements, each one slightly different according to the pitch and frequency of the sound being transmitted along the route, create nerve impulses which then travel to and along the auditory nerve to the brain where, finally, they are converted into recognisable sounds.[2] Quite breathtaking!

When we look at hearing in those with hEDS we need to start by considering a few interesting morphological issues which are often present. The earlobes are often really small (particularly in those hEDSers with a Marfan habitus) – earrings look delightful hanging from those sweet little lobes. The ear canals can be remarkably tiny and unusually angled. Earbuds are almost impossible to keep in as the teeny canals simply squeeze them out, and even the 'marshmallow' type either pop out or stay in but deform the soft surrounding tissues making hearing music impossible anyway. Not only can the eustachian tubes be a little 'floppy' but, as we will see, hypermobility of the jaw can also impact on secure eustachian tube function. Little wonder that many of us struggle with hearing issues and then struggle a second time trying to get information, support and appropriate treatment.

## Tinnitus

Tinnitus quite literally means 'ringing' in the ears, taken as it is from the Latin verb 'tinnire' which translates as 'to ring'.[3] Around 10 per cent of the population are described as suffering from tinnitus and about 5 per cent of those people are somewhat or very troubled by the condition. There are a variety of suspected causes for the condition and the sounds heard vary from person to person. Well-documented causes include hearing loss, medications, head injury and depression[4] – although depression itself can result from the distress and sleep loss caused by ongoing tinnitus. Amongst the many causes cited for tinnitus, in the hEDS population one possible culprit is temporomandibular joint dysfunction (TMJD) which, although a commonly described cause,[5] remains disputed.[6]

Whilst the hEDS client has an increased risk of developing TMJD,[7] which is explored below, more obviously and quite simply, with the increased laxity of connective tissue and cartilage, the ossicles within the middle ear can potentially move more than is ideal and lead to hearing disorders such as functional hearing loss and its noisy room mate, tinnitus.[8] Bafflingly, to my mind, trying to nail this all down is depressingly tough given that the relationship between hormonal laxity and tinnitus is described in both pregnancy and menopause but gets a rare passing mention in relation to hEDS.[9] It was left to my audiologist to explain why, unlike many tinnitus sufferers, for me, and for many hEDSers she and I speak to, white noise does not improve symptoms but actually leads to what I call 'competitive tinnitus' – the more noise that goes in, the louder the ringing and other tinnitus symptoms becomes. Those teeny bones moving more than they should amplify the vibrations and cause a confusing muddle of noise for the brain to work with.

Tinnitus can be exhausting – sometimes the ears just 'howl' with excess noise, allowing no moments of peace and whilst, for a large proportion of the general population, tinnitus is mild and occasional (particularly after a heavy night out), for those with clinically severe tinnitus it is relentless and so invasive that it can make conversations and watching TV miserable and even wake the sufferer up at night to bully them with yet more yelling.

Any condition that increases progesterone levels such as the pre-menstrual phase of a woman's cycle, pregnancy and menopause will impact on tissue laxity and increase the frequency and volume of a sufferer's tinnitus, and any medications that increase progesterone, such as the intrauterine coil, the mini and combined contraceptive pill and certain types of hormone replacement therapy (HRT), need to be prescribed with thought and care. Many other medications, including non-steroidal anti-inflammatories, are well known for increasing tinnitus,[10] which poses a real dilemma for people living with chronic pain *and* chronic tinnitus!

This hypermobility of the ossicles along with the hEDS effects on nerves (which we explored just a little in Chapter 4) may also be at the root of hearing loss.

*I started losing my hearing when I was 15–16. Finally, when my five-year-old was born and I was anxious about not hearing her, an otolar-yngologist took pity on me and did a wide range of tests. I won't ever forget his exclamation of 'I've never seen such flexible ear drums!' From perfect-pitch singer to hearing aids at age 34.*

Nicole

## Hearing Loss

Hearing seems to be a bit of a muddle for many with hEDS[11] and getting a diagnosis for the hearing distortions seems equally trying. Maybe conductive, maybe sensorineural, maybe functional? If the eustachian tubes are on the small and 'floppy' side then hearing loss might be very sporadic and, therefore, difficult to pin down, but that aside, something, somewhere along the line causes a greater than average number of people within the hEDS community to have hearing struggles of one sort or another and yet, many of us, when shut in a quiet box with a pair of headphones on and exposed to a series of beeps in the absence of any other distractions, perform relatively normally. The higher end of hearing is more often the part that can be picked up as mildly impaired due to conductive issues but an astonishing number of hEDSers I speak to have a diagnosis of 'functional hearing loss', which can translate loosely as 'You test normally and we have no idea why you say "pardon" all the time.' Google functional hearing loss and you will discover that this is often thought of as the 'you can hear what you want to hear' type of hearing, but this is to misunderstand the struggle that many of us describe.

Someone speaks and we hear quite well. We could also repeat what was said if given a few moments to think, but it's like our brain doesn't compute fast enough – like it's trying to translate from another language even though it does, in fact, know the language. And so there is that reflex 'pardon' whilst we wait for the penny to drop. And then, at other times, we really can't make it out. Busy environments with a lot of background noise in particular can be exhausting as we stare fixedly at the person talking to us waiting for our brain to sift through the melange and serve us up a morsel of clarity. When you consider how our brains are genuinely having to convert the rather over-cooked messages caused by somewhat erratic vibrations of the ossicles and imperfect nerve transmission you can see why we might not answer immediately. I realise that, on paper, this all sounds rather woolly (a bit like our hearing experience!) but there you have it.

## Temporomandibular Joint Dysfunction

Temporomandibular joint dysfunction (TMJD) is surprisingly common, affecting over 60 per cent of the adult population at one time or another.[12] Described as a condition affecting the temporomandibular joint and its surrounding muscles, it is generally short-lived and settles by itself. I suspect we have all experienced face-ache from having our mouth wide open in the dentist chair for a little too long. Our jaw aches and is stiff, our ears may hurt and we often get a headache to add to the mix. We have overstretched the joint at the base of our skull which joins our jaw to the rest of our head and allows for both side to side and up and down movements for talking and chewing. Once we have recovered from our time in the dentist chair, the TMJD disappears.

For around 5–12 per cent of the population, TMJ dysfunction is a chronic condition causing ongoing facial pain, earache, joint sounds in the TMJ such as clicking and grinding, difficulty opening the mouth, headaches, migraine, bruxism (tooth grinding) and sensitive teeth, pain and/or difficulty with chewing, and hearing disorders such as tinnitus.[13] Studies have demonstrated that between 50 per cent and 100 per cent of people with hEDS suffer with TMJ dysfunction and there is a significantly increased risk for recurrent (sometimes multiple times daily) TMJ dislocations.[14] It is useful to note that TMJD is more common where there is cranio-cervical instability and vice versa and that, along with the rest of the skeleton, the cervical spine in hEDS is more likely to be hypermobile, thereby exacerbating TMJD symptoms.[15] There is often a vicious circle set up with TMJ dysfunction – the pain causes teeth grinding and jaw clenching which, in turn, causes more pain in the TMJ and so on. Breaking that cycle can take time and, when there is a fundamental genetic issue creating the instability of the joint in the first place, getting any long-term relief from symptoms is a very tall order.

*I have TMJ dysfunction as diagnosed by the dentist, and have to be careful eating. I have subluxed my jaw several times by eating too much cake, or chocolate from the fridge!*

Alana

*My jaw is slightly misplaced so it clicks and I grind my teeth in my sleep, which gives me migraines (always a fun way to start the day!).*

Rosie

## Nose

Much more than just a sniffer out of smells, our nose also spends its time warming and moisturising the air we breathe before it hits the lungs, and filtering out inhaled pathogens and irritants (any that manage to bypass the system get reflexively sneezed out), thereby acting as our frontline defence system. The smell function of the nose, enabled by the inhaled air particles hitting the olfactory nerves, is closely aligned with taste, and any disruption to our sense of smell is likely to impact on our sense of taste. The spaces within the nose and facial bones (the sinuses) provide vocal resonance and aid clarity of speech.

### Deviated Nasal Septum

The shape of your nose is determined by your genetics, gender, internal cartilages and the septum, which is what divides our nose into two.[16] This cartilage is predominantly made up of collagen and is more likely to be deviated in those with connective tissue conditions, leading to congested breathing and sinusitis. A deviated septum, along with increased pharyngeal collapsibility due to tissue laxity, can give rise to a significantly increased likelihood of obstructive sleep apnoea so it is little wonder that hEDSers tend to be a snorey, sleep-deprived bunch.[17] Any increase in weight or tissue laxity will naturally exacerbate this condition and decrease quality of sleep even further.

### Rhinitis

Looking back to Chapter 3, you will remember that those with hEDS have an increased likelihood of allergy and atopy (including hay fever), and in Chapter 4 we saw how mast cell activity can be increased in the hEDS community. These factors, along with a deviated septum and fragile mucus membranes, mean that congestion can be a chronic problem, causing cough and rhinitis and further decreasing sleep quality.

## *Nosebleeds*

As we have seen in previous chapters, the more fragile mucous membranes in the nose are more likely to bleed. Nosebleeds without trauma are a common occurrence in those with any form of EDS,[18] particularly in childhood, and those with hEDS will often recount stories of spontaneous, prolonged nosebleeds alarming their friends and of even waking up smeared in blood when the nose has decided to bleed for no good reason during the night. My childhood friend can still remember me turning up on her doorstep, when my own parents were out, needing help with a nosebleed which seemed to go on for an eternity. It was a case of 'another day, another nosebleed' for me but she and her mum were genuinely shocked. Hormonal changes can make matters worse so that, by the time your pregnant hEDS client reaches your clinic, she might be alarmed by the return of her childhood bleeding episodes. Remember, this is not a platelet issue – it is a problem with the fragility of the capillary walls.

## Mouth and Throat

We explored the gastrointestinal system below the mouth and throat in the previous chapter, and also considered the lungs and respiratory system in Chapter 3, but now let's look at the upper respiratory tract and how swallowing and speech can be affected in those with hEDS.

We have seen how hiatus hernia, dysmotility, IBS and constipation are all increased in the hEDS population but, before food has even got that far, it has to make it out of the mouth and down the throat, and that is not as easy as it might sound when tissues are overstretchy and fragile and the nervous system is out of whack. The delicate, easily bruised tissues prevalent in hEDS mean that mouth ulcers are more common than in the general population and the gums may bleed more easily even with good dental hygiene.[19] The palate is often noticeably raised and overcrowding of the teeth is common[20] – there is frequently a history of tooth extraction in childhood to ease the overcrowding. There is a noticeable increase in abnormalities in both the lingual frenulum (the stretchy bit of skin under the tongue) and the labial frenulum (the stretchy bit of skin under the top lip), with some being absent[21] and some being unusually tight and posterior.[22]

It might be the lack of the lingual frenulum in some hEDSers which gives them the, frankly useless, ability to touch the tip of the nose with the tongue, a party trick known as Gorlin's sign whose only use is on those occasions when you have dipped down a little too deeply into your chocolate-sprinkled cappuccino and don't want to waste that sugary hit that is now decorating your deviated nasal septum!

## Dysphagia

The hypermobile tongue and temporomandibular joint can sometimes track a little erratically, which, along with the dysregulated autonomic nervous system (more about that in Chapter 8), can make swallowing a little hit and miss at times. Chewing and swallowing require a combination of chemical, mechanical and neurological messages to let our brain know that a swallow is needed. Then we need a coordinated jaw and tongue action along with correct breathing to make sure that the food or fluid goes down at the right time, into the right place, safely. That safety is achieved when, as we swallow, the food or fluid goes smoothly down the oesophagus into the stomach whilst the trachea is momentarily occluded. Sometimes, in hEDS, the timing all goes awry, synchronisation is lost and either there is gagging or the swallow simply won't trigger. It is the most bizarre sensation – you decide to swallow and...nothing. It is like your body cannot remember how to do it and you have to wait it out. Sometimes it goes part way and then the process seems to grind to a halt, giving a sensation of something being stuck in the throat. Sometimes there really is something stuck and it just goes down in its own sweet time, and at others, the throat simply has a bit of spasm giving the sensation of something being stuck – globus.[23] For most hEDSers this problem is a relatively mild, if occasionally alarming, issue but, for some, it is very life-affecting indeed and seriously impacts on their ability to eat normally.

## Voice Abnormalities

The voice is produced when air travels over the vocal folds (or cords), causing them to vibrate. Muscles attached to the larynx alter the tension within the cords, giving us the ability to alter pitch, whilst dynamic control is brought about through the use of the diaphragm and the speed and strength with which we push air over the cords. Whilst laxity in the cords and surrounding tissues might account for the finding that the EDS community has an unusually high proportion of accomplished singers, that same laxity can also lead to a variety of voice challenges. Dysphonia describes voice disturbance and can result in hoarseness or huskiness, vocal fatigue and voice loss in the absence of infection.[24] Professional singers are used to the experience of vocal fatigue and, in women, the monthly impact of changing hormones on their voice or the totally altered experience of voice production that pregnancy can cause – they drive their voices to work in a way that most of us cannot imagine. For those with hEDS the voice can tire with regular speaking and can fail completely mid-sentence without warning. Sometimes there is a sudden failure of the vocal cords to open at all, causing a brief but scary laryngospasm with an inability to breathe normally. Whilst this can happen in the daytime, due to the dysfunction of the hyper-mobile vocal cords, it can also happen at night, causing the unlucky sufferer to wake with a start, gasping for breath, heart pounding. Whilst the hormonal changes associated with the menstrual cycle, pregnancy and menopause can impact the voice of any woman, it is likely to be more marked in the hEDSer. The coughing, hoarseness and occasional laryngospasm may well be blamed on acid reflux and, whilst this can, of course, be the culprit (gastro-oesophageal reflux disease (GERD) being more common in the EDS population), vocal cord dysfunction should not be overlooked. Although the voice can tire easily, as with the rest of the EDS body, allowing it to become deconditioned through lack of exercise can cause more harm than good, leading to a downward spiral of symptoms. The 'use it or lose it' adage is essential advice for the hEDSer: they just need to be taught how to use it safely. The best prescription I was ever given was following a detailed laryngoscopy in the presence of an ENT doctor and a singing teacher to ascertain why I had suffered a sudden and total voice loss followed by prolonged huskiness. Having ruled out reflux and oesophagitis, I was put through my singing paces with a scope down my throat, after which I was told, 'When you sing, you control your vocal cords beautifully but when you talk, they are all over the place. We advise you to sing more!'

CHAPTER 6

# The Central
# Nervous System

## Introduction

We have been taking our guided tour around the body, studying each system in turn, and now we come to look at the system that ties it all together – the central nervous system (CNS). Without a functioning CNS and its co-worker, the peripheral nervous system (PNS), quite simply, nothing would happen – our limbs wouldn't move, our heart wouldn't beat, our food would remain undigested and we wouldn't even be able to think, or scheme or dream.

The CNS comprises the brain and spinal cord[1] whilst the peripheral nervous system is made up of the outer reaches of nerves, delivering and collecting information from limbs and organs and taking that back to the CNS.[2] The HQ of the CNS, quite literally the 'Head Honcho', is...the brain, which sits protected in the skull, and processes up to 11 million bits of information reaching it every second from all over the body. It then compresses that staggering amount of information down to less than 50 bits per second, which is what the conscious mind is apparently capable of dealing with,[3] although, frankly, before my second cup of coffee in the morning, my conscious brain can barely cope with remembering my own name!

The spinal cord descends from the medulla oblongata at the base of the brain to between the second and third lumbar vertebrae. Here it spreads out into the cauda equina and off into the peripheral nervous system. The spinal cord is protected on the outside by the bones, muscles and tendons of the vertebral column as well as by three protective layer of tissue – the meninges. It is bathed and cushioned outside and in by the cerebrospinal fluid (CSF).

Information is transmitted along nerves by a complex electrochemical process which relies for its efficacy on the cord being able to move and stretch just the right amount...

There is a significant body of evidence pointing to numerous effects on all parts of the nervous system caused by EDS and it appears that, in the case of the CNS, many of the symptoms arriving on the desk of physicians seeing EDS clients are caused by overstretching of the spinal cord leading to disruption of the electrochemical transmission process as well as short- and long-term injury.

# Headache

Entire books have been written on the subject of headaches and there won't be an adult alive who has not, at some point, experienced one. Those with EDS suffer with headache more than most, and those with hEDS and vEDS more than other EDS subtypes.[4] Migraine (with or without aura) is much more common, tends to be of earlier onset, occurs more frequently and is of a more severe nature in those with hEDS than in the general population.[5] With more than 150 causes of headache across the whole population, the hEDS client is likely to have both 'normal' and hEDS-related headaches, and it can be difficult for them to sift out the 'normal' headache wheat from the hEDS-related chaff. Let's examine the various ways in which hEDS can cause and exacerbate headache:

## *Cranio-cervical Instability*

The most mobile part of the spine is at the cranio-cervical junction, where the neck meets the head.[6] The human head is heavy and, for the hEDSer, fighting 24/7 to 'hold it all together', it can feel *really* heavy. The average UK baby weighs in at 3.5kg and the average human head weighs about 5kg, and the cranio-cervical joint has been described as being like balancing a bowling ball on the top of a pencil. There are ample muscles, tendons and ligaments all working hard to ensure good stability in the neck but, if the cranio-cervical junction is lax then the head really can wobble about, stretching the spinal cord and causing an array of acute and chronic symptoms as well as long-term damage to the vertebral discs, leading to early disc degeneration.[7]

Headache triggered by cranio-cervical instability (CCI) can take the form of migraine, daily persistent headache, cervicogenic headache, neck-tongue syndrome and, given that the cranio-cervical junction and temporomandibular joint work so closely together, TMJ dysfunction. Even on days when the headache is not severe, there can be a constant dull headache humming away in the background. If an hEDS client seeks help with their persistent head pain and is sent for radiological studies, chances are that they will be laid down for the imaging and, needless to say, results will show no abnormality of the spinal cord – the problem will only show when the head is in flexion or extension such as when standing.[8]

Treating headache caused by CCI is hard – interventions such as diet modification, pain medications, relieving stress and so on do not alter the genetics and the hEDSer still has to attempt to hold her head up and in the right position whilst she goes about her everyday life, hampered as she is by a lack of proprioception. Something as simple as turning the head quickly to see where a noise is coming from, or braking a little over-enthusiastically when driving might cause the head to move too far out of the normal range, overstretch the spinal cord and trigger the onset of a severe headache. A headache brought on by a sudden over-extension of the cranio-cervical junction can come on unbelievably fast and spread up the neck, across through the teeth and up into the face and head and quickly become quite incapacitating – I have had to pull over in my car when I have triggered one, such was the speed and intensity of the onset.

*Cranio-cervical instability: I believe I'm so used to the struggles that it makes me fantastic at masking. I can be stuck in bed all day with pain, from doing something as simple as trying to lift my bag up from the floor to the bed while I'm sitting on the bed.*

Michelle

## Atlantoaxial Instability

The conjoined twin to CCI, atlantoaxial instability refers specifically to the alignment of the top two vertebrae in the cervical spine (C1 and C2), the atlantoaxial junction (AAJ), which is the single most mobile joint of the body.[9] Instability of this joint can cause intense neck and occipital pain and, because the abnormal movement of this joint can affect blood flow, there may be visual changes, pre-syncope or syncope (feeling faint or actually fainting), dizziness and nausea. The joint can be very tender to touch and there might be facial pain and difficulties with swallowing. Because CCI and atlantoaxial instability are so closely related, the terms are often used interchangeably.

## Chiari Malformation

The base of the brain, the cerebellum, normally sits within the skull just above the opening (foramen magnum) leading to the spinal cord below. In Chiari malformation, the very lowest part of the cerebellum, known as the tonsils, herniates through the base of the skull and the resulting pressure around them causes an array of symptoms.[10] The condition is generally present from birth due to a birth defect, and may or may not be associated with hydrocephalus but often doesn't present symptomatically until the teenage years. The prevalence of Chiari used to be considered to be around 1 in 1000 but, with the growth in the use of good brain imaging, it is now thought possible it could be nearer to 1 in 100 births. It is not certain as to whether EDS, with its increased likelihood of prolapse, has a causal or correlative relationship with Chiari but it seems as if the increased cranio-cervical instability might give rise to Chiari symptoms even when the cerebral tonsils are only very mildly herniated and might not otherwise cause symptoms.[11]

The symptoms associated with Chiari are caused by the pressure of the herniated tonsils occupying the foramen magnum interfering with circulation of cerebrospinal fluid,[12] and this might provide the clue as to why some with hEDS have Chiari symptoms with minimal to no herniation of the cerebral tonsils – that cranio-cervical instability giving rise to hyper-extension and flexion of the head, settling of the head down onto the spine at the cranio-cervical joint, and a subsequent interference with CSF circulation.

Symptoms are multiple and varied: headache – particularly occipital and triggered by coughing and Valsalva (yet one more reason to encourage client-led pushing in second stage of labour), blurred vision, intolerance of movement, tinnitus, clumsiness, speech problems, autonomic dysfunction, sleep disorders, chronic fatigue and altered pain perception. Now, of course, many of these symptoms are often present in hEDS anyway and there may be no Chiari but, as with imaging of the cranio-cervical joint, radiological investigations are generally done with the patient lying down, when the problem isn't obvious, so it is very difficult to know the true extent of Chiari malformation in the symptomatic hEDS client. The symptomatic client with no visible Chiari malformation on MRI might be given a diagnosis of Chiari malformation type 0 or of cervical medullary syndrome – all the symptoms but without a visible cause.

Having explored headache in hEDS, let's move on to other impacts of the condition on the CNS.

## Tethered Cord Syndrome

In normal anatomy, the spinal cord hangs quite loosely within the spinal column, allowing it to move when its owner bends, stretches or grows. It is given just enough stability by a fine strand of fibrous tissue called the filum terminale, which attaches to the dura mater at the very base of the vertebral column. Tethered cord syndrome (TCS) describes a condition whereby the end of the cord is attached too much or held too tightly by the surrounding tissues. The limit to free movement of the cord that this tethering can cause can result in a range of symptoms – pain in the lower back, buttocks and perineum, muscle weakness, loss of sensation in the legs and feet, and bladder and bowel dysfunction. It seems that TCS in the hEDS community might present a little differently – the symptoms might be more episodic rather than constant, and headache, sub-occipital and neck pain are more likely to be seen as a symptom compared to those diagnosed with TCS but who do *not* also have hEDS. There also seems to be a different mechanism at play, with the culprit in hEDS appearing to be the stress on the fragile and overstretchy tissues causing micro-damage to the fibres of the filum terminale[13] rather than there being a radiologically demonstrable over-tethering of the cord. As with cranio-cervical instability, the inability to find the problem in the radiology department can put an obstacle in the way of the hEDSer searching for answers to their symptoms.

## Degenerative Disc Disease/Spondylosis

Backs take a heck of a lot of punishment through life – those 33 little vertebral bones, separated by their protective, cushioning discs and supported by their surrounding muscles and ligaments, give us a spine which can bend and stretch in pretty much any direction at the same time as protecting the most important nerves we possess. Imagine trying to get through your day without that flexible rod allowing you to tie your laces, play sport, reach to the top shelf or even check over your shoulder when you drive. So it is no surprise that with age often comes degeneration of the discs,[14] weakening of the ligaments, arthritis of the vertebrae and the subsequent smorgasbord of neck and back pain, pain radiating down the buttocks, and numbness and tingling in the arms and legs which sometimes comes with a loss in strength and movement – you know how your nan struggles with doing up buttons and other fine motor skills? A bit of hand arthritis maybe, but probably also some age-related degenerative disc disease (DDD). This array of DDD symptoms is also called myelopathy, and at the more severe end of the scale also includes unsteady gait, loss of balance and, when the cauda equina is impacted, loss of normal bladder and bowel function. This symptomatic degeneration of the vertebral column, although part of the ageing process, affects women more commonly than men,[15] and the course of the disease is speeded up by excess weight gain and repetitive strain to the spine.

The hEDS spine is on an accelerated journey towards this relatively common consequence of ageing, with early-onset DDD being well documented.[16] The vertebrae being so much freer to move, and to move too far, can not only damage the collagen-rich discs more easily but can also allow for a greater likelihood of disc herniation. The discs, once injured, are slower to heal and, living in an hEDS body, as fast as they do heal, are subjected to yet more stress and injury. Your pregnant hEDS client has the whole female, weight-gain, repetitive strain bonanza to offer as a gift to her already overstrained spine and, once her baby is born, she is not going to have any less weight-bearing to do – that baby is only going to get heavier – have a less hypermobile spine, or get any younger!

## Pain

Of course, we have already explored the pain associated with hEDS at pretty much every point so far but, as we consider the CNS, it is vital to think about the way this population experiences pain and why. All humans experience pain – we fall over, or bang our head, or catch the top of the oven as we reach in to grab that delicious tray of freshly baked biscuits and...it hurts! No surprises there. Nor would it surprise anyone to know that more frequent injuries lead to more frequent pain experiences. But something else goes on in the hEDS body which causes a paradoxical situation whereby there can be an increase in chronic pain in particular, whilst the hypermobility reduces with ageing, and there is sometimes intense pain felt long after an injury has healed and in the absence of any demonstrable pathology. The younger hEDSer typically experiences the acute pain of injury – that twisted ankle sustained through a combination of poor proprioception and wobbly joints – but, as the years go on, the pain can become widespread, difficult to locate, deep and unremitting with nothing to show on X-ray or MRI. So what is going on?

Head back to Chapter 4 on the GI system and you will remember that the nerves themselves contain collagen and the surrounding tissue is more yielding, which allows them to be more easily aggravated. Then, at the start of the present chapter we saw how information is sent along the nerves using an electrochemical process that is tied in with the stretching and moving of the spinal cord. At the level of the brain there is the potential for complete overwhelm as it tries to do what every brain does whilst having the additional work of trying to stay upright, keep the blood pumping effectively around a rather too soft circulatory system, deal with an overly emotional gut, try to clarify the somewhat chaotic audio messages, manage the pain of acute injury and generally keep the whole show on the road. It is in a permanently hypervigilant state of arousal. Something has to go on the back burner and that something is those moment-by-moment micro-injuries caused by joints and muscles continually moving out of their normal healthy range: tiny tears to the abnormally soft connective tissues and almost imperceptible bruises as insignificant bumps cause the more delicate capillaries to fracture. The brain just puts up barriers to that information and decides to leave all that till later...

One day, there is the straw that breaks the hEDS camel's back and it can be something fairly insignificant – an everyday sort of sprain, or a bout of flu – and those carefully constructed barriers, put up to keep the huge mass of daily 'trivial' micro-traumas at bay, come crashing down and then there is bedlam. Suddenly the brain 'sees' all those old micro-injuries it has steadfastly ignored and, even though they are now long recovered, it starts feeling and obsessing with them. The only way I have satisfactorily found to explain it is by calling it pain or nerve tinnitus. This is just background noise with no real meaning except that which the brain decides to confer on it but, as with tinnitus, the brain won't switch its attention away from the noise to let it disappear into the background again. Imagine a whole lifetime of injury in every part of your body all coming into focus at once and you'll have some idea of how a flare can feel, and the first event can be terrifying. Unlike the regular pain of injury that hEDSers live with from their earliest days, this presents a unique challenge – widespread, intractable pain, often along with flu-like symptoms, and no discernible pathology. So we get sent to bed to rest and our bodies which rely on regular exercise to remain conditioned and less painful, get worse...fast. Rest, opiates and being hypervigilant about pain because 'pain is the body's way of telling you there is a problem' can all make the day-to-day pain of hEDS worse.[17]

hEDSers talk about their 'flares' and experience them in a variety of ways. Alongside the sudden onset of widespread pain, there might also be an increase in subluxing or popping joints – things get more 'slidey', brain fog can descend, dysautonomia can increase, GI symptoms worsen...it's miserable.

*The dysautonomia I developed as a result of my many injuries and operations was some of the worst pain I have ever experienced. Objectively my foot was fine, but my nerve system seemed to think there was something that needed pain signalling.*

Nadia

*Don't mistake my positivity as a sign that I'm OK. I have widespread pain on a daily basis, mostly due to my dislocations, but I am the most*

*positive person and I think this often is the reason medical professionals*
*assume that I'm OK. When really I'm not.*

Faye

I remember my worst ever flare. I cannot remember the trigger but I think I had, quite simply, sat too long with my foot bent at an unhelpful angle whilst I was watching TV. Within 24 hours I was in such considerable pain, worst in my ankle but all over my body, to a degree that when it was still giving me vivid nightmares and waking me yelling some weeks later, I was assessed for bone cancer and sent for bed rest whilst I waited, terrified, for results. By the time my results showed that I was making a big old fuss about nothing, I was needing orthotic splints and long rehabilitation with a physiotherapist. Once I started to accept that the pain was an echo of all my previous injuries which my brain had hooked on to and couldn't resist checking in on, I learnt to relax into it, exercise in spite of the pain, meditate on the pain and allow it just to ease into the background again.

No obvious pathology, everything hurts, fluey feelings and understandable exhaustion and intolerance to exercise? You won't find many hEDSers who haven't been diagnosed with fibromyalgia and/or myalgic encephalomyelitis/chronic fatigue syndrome (ME/CFS) and consequently had correct diagnosis and appropriate support and treatment delayed by years or decades. Of course, as with every other population, those with hEDS can also be struck by fibromyalgia and ME, and people with these conditions might also be part of the hEDS community, but the conditions are different and some of the appropriate treatments for one condition may be harmful if used to treat another.[18]

For very many women living with hEDS, there is a common camel-breaking straw: a critical time when their super-stretchy, over-alerted body gets such a massive increase in joint stress that it can spill over and trigger a flare like no other – pregnancy. And this woman is walking into your clinic!

## CHAPTER 7

# Genitourinary Systems

## Introduction

The genitourinary system is also known as the urinogenital system…and then there is the professional speciality of urogynaecology to confuse matters even further. With my years as a midwife, I'm more inclined to use 'genitourinary' as a term and so, forgive me, I am sticking to my guns!

The literature on this part of the hEDS-affected body is as frustratingly muddled as that for the other systems – often the studies are small and that's to be expected when studying a small subset of the population. But when all the various types of EDS are sometimes lumped together and sometimes taken separately all in the same paper, it can make it tricky to know what's what. Sometimes the best we can do is simply say, 'This may or may not be likely to affect your hEDS client, so keep your wits about you!'

## Urinary System

Consisting of the kidneys, ureters, bladder and urethra, the urinary system does more than simply keep us acquainted with the smallest room in the house. Through its elimination of excess fluid from the body, blood pressure, blood pH and blood volume are all regulated, and the correct electrolyte and mineral balance is maintained.[1]

The kidneys are the filtration unit of the body, and just over a litre of blood passes through the two of them for sprucing up every minute, resulting in an average daily urine output of between one and two litres depending on activity, hydration and the environment. The urine flows into the bladder through the ureters where it is stored until its human owner has made it to the loo, locked out a curious cat (hasn't it heard about the terminal impact of curiosity to felines?) and four demanding kids, fought through the nightmare of over-engineered clothes and finally relaxed enough to consciously 'let it all out'...or is that just my house?

The urinary system is lined with a unique type of transitional epithelium called uroepithelium, which has distensibility as its super-power. The smooth muscle of the bladder is fascinating. Think about it – when you stress any other muscle in the body, it contracts. But stress the bladder by filling it and...it relaxes. And then, when you relax and make a conscious decision to pee, it goes into spasm. Genius. Ever wondered why kids all instinctively know the 'I need a wee dance'? They discover that, when they need a wee but their Lego® is way more interesting, they stress the bladder by jiggling around and it relaxes a little, enabling them to play a tiny bit longer. They dance and so they really 'don't need to go now'! Then, of course, they relax and... whoops – better get that mop!

The muscle at the heart of this smart little design is the detrusor, and it takes a while to develop its knack, which is why babies need nappies or a parent's lap until they are old enough to be able to learn to spot the signals and either hang on or empty. There are also hormones involved in the production and concentration of urine, particularly vasopressin (also know as anti-diuretic hormone), which is produced in a circadian rhythm and is responsible for concentrating the urine more overnight, thereby reducing the need to pee when you could be knocking out the zeds.

So, because of the unique distensibility of the bladder tissue there is no increase in pressure as it fills and so the human is able to hold, on average, nearly half a litre of urine quite comfortably. Eventually though, a limit is reached and pain receptors are activated and we feel the need to pee. Ignore that urge and it can quickly start to be very uncomfortable even though the volume inside the bladder might not have increased by more than a few tablespoons. What enables us to keep hanging on until safely locked away in private are the internal and external urethral sphincters.[2] The internal sphincter, in particular, deserves a medal as it remains constantly squeezed, in the face of all bladder-stretching odds, until conscious voiding is activated, thanks to its modified striated muscle. Once we decide to pee, the internal sphincter allows urine out of the bladder and then the external sphincter enables us to control the power and speed of the flow as we let the pee hit the pan.

When subjected to the multitudinous delights of hEDS, this fabulous little system can start to creak, and leak, at the seams...

## Urinary Incontinence

Getting accurate data on the incidence of urinary incontinence in women is tricky – so many confounders around age, weight, parity and lifestyle – but a meta-analysis of studies suggests that somewhere between about 13 per cent and 46 per cent of female adults in the general population have some urinary incontinence (defined as unintended passing of urine);[3] the incidence is lower in younger women and then goes up with age. Incidence is higher in women who have given birth at least once, although having more babies doesn't appear to make matters worse until you get to your fourth birth.[4] Take a look at the stats for those with hEDS and there is a marked difference, with almost 70 per cent in one study complaining of incontinence, compared to an incidence in a control group of women without hEDS of 30 per cent,[5] and similar doubling of figures found across other studies.

It would be easy to assume that the cause for this significant incidence of urinary incontinence in the hEDS population is rather stretchy and incompetent urethral sphincters failing to prevent leakage but, although this can certainly be true, this doesn't explain quite a lot of the incontinence cases. To understand things a little better we need to consider the different types of urinary incontinence.

When broken down into subsets we find that sometimes people leak when they cough, laugh or lift something heavy. This is stress incontinence. Some people don't leak at all when they cough or sneeze but will suddenly feel the need to go and then can't make it to the loo in time. This is called urinary urgency or urge incontinence. Sometimes both of these types of incontinence are present in the same person (mixed urinary incontinence). Finally, there is overflow incontinence which is exactly what is says on the can – the bladder gets over-full without being able to empty and then it all gets too much and it simply cannot fill any more, the urethral sphincters give up their struggle to stay closed and the inevitable gush occurs.

## Stress Incontinence

With stress incontinence, the pressure inside the bladder, increased with a cough, sneeze, laugh, etc., overcomes the urethral sphincter pressure and so urine escapes. There isn't a bladder contraction in this case. This type of incontinence generally occurs as a result of muscle or sphincter nerve damage or incompetence due to surgery or childbirth (particularly where there is a prolonged or precipitate second stage), loss of vaginal tissue tone (vaginal atrophy) in menopause, and chronic cough or constipation. The hEDS population is more susceptible to stress incontinence as a result of their lax collagen fibres, and, whereas stress incontinence is rarely seen in the general nulliparous, pre-menopausal population, it can certainly affect those with hEDS who have never had children and are not yet menopausal.[6] However, it appears that the considerably higher rates of incontinence may actually be due to a different cause altogether…

## Urinary Urgency

This type of incontinence is different. Whereas with stress incontinence there is an element of anticipation – 'I'm going to sneeze, so better squeeze!' – with urgency there is no warning. Quite simply, the detrusor muscle goes into overdrive and the bladder contracts without warning and whether or not there is a full bladder. Suddenly there is a desperate need to pee but…too late already! Sometimes called an 'overactive bladder', the main causes of this miserable affliction are increased sensitivity to the neurotransmitter acetylcholine which causes the smooth muscle of the detrusor to contract, and irritation of the bladder due to drugs, foods, infection and inflammation.

Now, despite the reasonable assumption that all incontinence in the hEDS population must be stress incontinence due to weak collagen lending poor support to the urethra, it seems that there may actually be significantly more detrusor overactivity, with over 62 per cent incidence of urgency incontinence in the hEDS community compared to 38 per cent with the non-hEDS population.[7] There appear to be a few factors at work – there is over double the rate of urinary tract infections, nearly triple the number suffering from bladder pain and incomplete bladder emptying and nearly four times the risk of having problems in actually consciously peeing. Looking in more detail, the hEDS bladder seems to have more mast cells in the muscle tissue and the body over-reacts to having a urinary tract infection (UTI) and causes inflammation which, in turn, can lead to more UTIs[8] and continue to cause symptoms but without necessarily triggering a positive urinalysis (dipstick) test in the consulting room.[9] So, fundamentally, something more immunological seems to be happening with the overactive bladder in this population.

## *Overflow Incontinence*

Whilst some with hEDS suffer with irritable bladders, constantly struggling with a low-grade UTI, bladder pain and an over-enthusiastic detrusor muscle, there are those whose hyper-stretchy bladder simply fills and fills with no increase in the internal bladder pressure which would see most people desperately dashing to the loo.[10] The pressure doesn't rise, the pain receptors aren't triggered and nobody is any the wiser. When you couple this with the fact that, in order to maintain stability in that bendy body, many hEDSers keep their pelvic floor muscles almost permanently switched on which, in turn, can lead to the urethral sphincters being over-engaged, it is no surprise that a subset of those with hEDS simply don't get the memo that their bladder is filling up. But, even with the stretchiest bladders, there is a limit and, when this huge-capacity bladder gives up its load...close the Thames Barrier! For these women, with their super-strong pelvic floors and sphincters, when they do make it to the loo in good time (maybe using a clock rather than internal signals as a guide) they might have to actively strain to pee. I confess to being part of this group and can hold on, completely without any discomfort, all day...even when pregnant! I am happy to say that I manage to go before it's too late by listening in to other signals (trousers a little tight!) and I make a damned fine hiking companion who will never keep you waiting whilst I hunt around for a good place to pee every couple of hours. My husband is a mere mortal when it comes to bladder capacity and cannot fathom why I simply don't get the concept of an 'insurance wee'!

> *My bladder is like a balloon and can hold almost two litres! I have to self-cath to remove all the wee as my bladder muscles can't contract. I have painful, long, heavy periods and am not able to take many forms of contraception.*

> Hana

## Gynae System

So what about the genito- side of the genitourinary system? Well, as with the urinary side of things, the evidence is somewhat mixed, and confused by the conflation of the different subtypes, but it is quite clear that those with hEDS suffer as a result of their fragile, overstretchy tissues and their bodies' constantly over-alerted state of being.

### Pain

The reduced protection of nerves due to the lack of firm, structured tissue around them along with the dysfunction in the way messages seem to travel along the nerve fibres, and the fragility of the tissues, means that those with hEDS complain far more than the general population about gynaecological pain. From dyspareunia (painful sex), to vulvodynia and vulva vestibulitis (vulval pain and inflammation) through to dysmenorrhea (painful periods),[11] this population can really suffer. One study found over 60 per cent of women with hEDS suffering from dyspareunia[12] which, for a population already hampered by generalised pain and anxiety and struggling to shake off a label of neurotic hypochondriac, really can feel like the last straw – just when you've found a position where your hips don't sublux you discover that even the slightest of intimate touches feel like fire, and not in a good way! With so much ongoing shame and secrecy about periods and sex along with societal and cultural assumptions surrounding women's experience of pain as just 'part of being a woman', this aspect of hEDS life gets very little airing, leaving many feeling isolated and scared.

> *I've experienced vulvodynia off and on over 20 years now but pregnancy and the additional blood flow and sensitivity just tipped me over the edge. It was fire.*
>
> Nina

### Bleeding

As women we get used to the fascinating rhythms and swinging of our oestrogen–progesterone balance and the shedding of the endometrium which accompanies each menstrual cycle. It has been noted that those with hEDS are more likely to be sensitive to these hormonal fluctuations,[13] making them more susceptible to pre-menstrual tension (PMT), intolerance to hormonal contraceptives, and menorrhagia (heavy periods) as well as the hormonal changes that mark pregnancy and the puerperium. Heavy bleeding during menstruation is stated in one study to affect around 30 per cent of all women in their reproductive years[14] but the National Institute for Health and Care Excellence (NICE) guidance finds less than 5 per cent of women consult their doctor with heavy menses.[15] Given that the NICE publication also states that around 20 per cent of women aged under 60 have a hysterectomy, often for heavy bleeding, it seems clear that many women are suffering their menorrhagia in silence.

*I could not tolerate hormones at all. I tried several combination pills and the mini pill. By far the worst side effect was the psychological harm. With no history of mental health issues, I was suddenly suffering from severe depression and unable to get out of bed.*

Kathy

It's very hard for women themselves to judge whether or not their bleeding is abnormally heavy because, unless they're a midwife or otherwise 'in the business', they simply don't get to see the monthly blood loss of other women. Heavy loss is generally defined as more than a measured loss of 80cl during the cycle. Measured loss? Sheesh!

Anyway, between 50 per cent and 75 per cent of women with hEDS complain of menorrhagia,[16] which, by any measurement, is significantly more than the general population. Whether this is due to the increased fragility of the tissues as the endometrium sheds, the increased sensitivity to circulating and fluctuating hormones or a combination of both is unclear but I suspect, from my own experience and that of many of my clients, and from conversations with my own specialist doctor, that it is the latter.

Aside from the impact on menses, the fragility of tissues leading to bleeding can impact on sex life, the wearing of less-than-super-soft sanitary towels, pubic shaving, and even going to the toilet – wiping after going to the loo really can cause bleeding of the delicate hEDS vulval mucosa, and I triggered quite a discussion when I asked on an

EDS forum about the best toilet paper to use – spoiler alert: forget loo paper and get a bidet!

It must be stressed again that there really aren't platelet or other clotting abnormalities in hEDS, simply fragile tissues and blood cell walls. The sensitivity to hormonal activity might also account for the increased incidence of dysmenorrhea – the uterus reacting more strongly to the tocolytic action of prostaglandins as the endometrium is shed. We shall consider this again when looking at the third stage of birth in Chapter 15. This experience of intense pain and bleeding can have a mixed impact on those considering pregnancy – will they be more able to cope with the pain and blood loss of birth, or frightened at the prospect of yet more pain in their life when they feel they've endured enough?

## Endometriosis

I hear a lot in the hEDS community about a potential association with endometriosis but there is currently scant and very mixed evidence for this.[17] Maybe the increased incidence in the hEDS population of increased pain and heavy bleeding has led to this question being raised. In any event, I add this in because, with a bit of luck, by the time you're reading this, more studies will have been conducted and you'll be ahead of the game!

## Prolapse

Again, the evidence for pelvic organ prolapse (POP) in the hEDS population is very mixed due to the paucity of studies which don't lump all subtypes together. But overall, studies seem to support the view that there is an increased risk of POP in the more bendy members of our society.[18]

Pelvic organ prolapse can affect the uterus, the vagina and the bladder, causing a feeling of heaviness around the lower tummy and genitals, dragging sensations and a sense of something coming down inside the vagina, dyspareunia (seriously, it's a wonder hEDSers ever have any fun under the duvet) and problems peeing. Maintaining a healthy weight, avoiding lifting heavy objects and reducing the likelihood of constipation are essential strategies in avoiding and managing

POP, but when your body appears to be intent on ignoring all your efforts to firm and tighten up, action plans can feel pretty dispiriting.

## Miscarriage

For those with hEDS who either don't have or who can overcome the often excruciating pain of vulvodynia or vulva vestibulitis, and who are otherwise healthy in spite of everything their body can throw at them, there is then the hurdle of getting and staying pregnant. Those with the classic subtype are very much more at risk of both early and late miscarriage but those in the hypermobile subtype may also be more at risk, although the evidence is mixed. Around 20 per cent of all pregnancies end in miscarriage[19] and, of course, this number includes those with hEDS. Within the hEDS population alone the risk has been quoted as nearer 28 per cent,[20] with a significantly higher than average risk of multiple miscarriage (13%[21] against 1% in the overall population[22]). It would be easy to blame this apparent increased risk on incompetency of the cervix due to lax tissue structure but, given that the risk of premature birth is no greater than average in those with hEDS,[23] I suspect that we should be more focused on remembering that this is a population who may well be poorly nourished, often on a plethora of medications and, where mobility is restricted, potentially carrying significant excess weight. For those with hEDS who have managed to create a healthy lifestyle and limited their use of medication, one would hope that the risk of miscarriage is reduced to nearer that of the general population. Certainly other studies have not shown an increased risk of miscarriage in the hEDS population[24] and, where there is miscarriage, it has not been shown to be resulting from the condition. The messages, as so often is the case with this condition, are very mixed.

Suffice to say that the hEDSer coming your way likely brings with her a long and sorry history of incontinence, pelvic pain and heavy vaginal bleeding and, as we will see in the next chapter, even in the unlikely absence of all this, the woman in front of you is prone to huge anxiety!

## CHAPTER 8

# The Autonomic Nervous System

## Introduction

Finally, to the autonomic nervous system. I have left this part until last because, although out there in the shop window on full display are those long, bendy limbs, popping joints, bruises, gut issues and the plethora of other obvious, physical manifestations of hEDS, for those living with the condition, it is often the more hidden aspects of this connective tissue syndrome which can drag them down day to day. The impact on the ANS can also be the one area which, when they try to explain it, leaves other people scratching their head – they can understand IBS and muscle pain and nasty bruises, but the dysregulation of the ANS takes us into the dark arts area of EDS where things get seriously weird. There is always a sense of huge relief to meet another hEDSer who doesn't look suspicious when you say, 'I'm having one of those days when I keep forgetting to breathe!' I told you things here get weird...

The autonomic nervous system is a subdivision of the peripheral nervous system and is itself subdivided into the sympathetic and parasympathetic systems – sometimes described as like the accelerator and brake working in opposition to maintain functional stability and respond to stress. The ANS governs those bodily functions outside conscious control, including heart rate, breathing, thermoregulation, blood pressure and certain reflex actions such as coughing, sneezing, swallowing and vomiting. It is the sympathetic division of the ANS that controls the 'flight or fight' response and homeostasis as the 'accelerator', and the parasympathetic division that is involved with the slower, 'brake' side of things such as sleep and digestion.[1]

The volume and range of management that is the bread and butter of the ANS is simply staggering and cannot be covered here, but just consider how much happens within your body without your conscious effort – sure there is breathing and swallowing but what about the regulation of blood sugar, or sweating, or the secretion of saliva? We simply take the day-to-day background unconscious running of our body for granted...until it goes wrong!

The ANS in all subtypes of EDS tends to be dysregulated, but the hEDS population is more affected than the other subtypes,[2] with up to 80 per cent of hEDSers experiencing symptoms.[3] The exact mechanism around its failure to work normally is not understood but what is certain is that there is rather an over-exaggerated response to internal triggers so that relatively weak stimuli (maybe a slight drop in blood sugar) are 'seen' by the ANS as a big old nose-dive and the hEDSer looks and feels for all the world as if they are properly hypoglycaemic. Naturally, their blood checks say 'nothing to see here!' This over-enthusiastic response can lead to an over-correction, then another over-response, and it's all pretty chaotic.

## Postural Orthostatic Tachycardia Syndrome

The overriding diagnosis that is given to this ANS dysregulation is postural orthostatic tachycardic syndrome (POTS), which we met briefly in Chapter 3 on the cardiovascular system. You'll remember that this is generally defined by its owner's inability to tolerate changes to posture – the pulse rises significantly (by more than 30 beats per minute) on sitting up or standing, and there is sometimes, but not always, an accompanying drop in blood pressure.[4] We will look at this feature in detail but it is important to realise that this POT bit of the picture simply describes a part of the whole syndrome – the S in POTS. Many with hEDS will not suffer greatly with the POT part but will really struggle with the S bit, which encompasses all the other ANS elements. If a client says she has POTS, therefore, it is unwise to assume that she is describing feeling faint and nauseous when getting up. She might do, but she might be far more troubled by her poor thermoregulation, or her digestive shenanigans.

First named in 1993[5] and then formally defined in 2011,[6] the orthostatic tachycardia aspect of POTS demonstrates the over-responsiveness of the ANS in all its glory. The client gets the head rush to end all head rushes as they sit up, stand or, sometimes, just move their head a little too quickly, and often feels nauseous and as if they are going to faint. But they generally don't. In the normal course of events in the general population, on standing up, there is a measurable increase in heart rate and then the ANS quickly adjusts back to normal. Job done! In POTS the ANS, sensing the change in posture, overcompensates, sending the heart rate right up, and then over-adjusts again, sending it back down, then up and then down in a ridiculous panicky ANS equivalent of running round like a headless chicken.[7] The unlucky client might feel like fainting, but often doesn't because the body keeps adjusting before the faint happens, only for it to cycle back to pre-syncope again.[8] No wonder this is so often accompanied by nausea.

The condition can be debilitating and catch the sufferer in quite the vicious cycle – exercise is one of the fundamental parts of management but how can someone exercise when they feel faint and sick just getting up? So they become very deconditioned and more and more fearful of doing something which would help to reduce their symptoms. Maintaining good hydration by taking regular fluids and salts can help to stabilise blood pressure and for those most seriously affected, a range of medications can be tried. Even those hEDSers who are not debilitated by the orthostatic tachycardia generally recognise and share the symptoms on a less grand scale. Every human recognises the symptoms of head rush, but for those with hEDS it can hit after the slightest motion and hang around and rush in and out for a lot longer. If it's a bad day or at a certain point in the menstrual cycle then this cycling of the ANS as it goes into overdrive can cause repeated mini-attacks for hours on end, sending the hEDSer constantly rummaging through her supply of salty snacks and chugging back the isotonic drinks in an attempt to reach equilibrium.

## Thermoregulation

I have yet to meet someone with hEDS who does not have issues with thermoregulation. Women operate within a narrower band than men when it comes to temperature comfort[9] and so this is one of those big 'me too' areas I mentioned at the very start of the first chapter.

Whereas the average woman might complain of 'always' having cold hands and feet, when her ANS realises that she is chilly, it does all the right things to rectify the situation and, as long as she hauls on an extra jumper, she'll start to feel more comfortable. Basically, that jumper is used to hold in the heat that she is making and her ANS will regulate her temperature, keeping her comfy once she has reached the right level. Also, the non-hEDS woman will correctly sense her internal temperature – she will feel what she really is, temperature-wise.

The hEDSer simply doesn't function like that – just like a baby who is incapable of normal thermoregulation and requires a radiating heat source (a lovely bit of skin to skin with its parent), so it is with those with hEDS. Irregularities in shivering and sweating can result in a situation where the woman with hEDS feels very cold, and all those extra jumpers will simply trap in the cold because her thermostat is faulty. Remember also that, because of the inability of the nerves to transmit bodily sensations correctly, this woman might feel freezing cold even though her skin might feel warm enough and her measured temperature will likely read within a normal range. In order to warm up properly, she needs that radiating heat source, so she snuggles into her partner or trusty hot water bottle. Then, all of a sudden, the ANS swings into action, all guns blazing, but over-eggs the pudding somewhat and now she feels so hot it's claustrophobic, and she can't cool down. She fights free from her beloved who just five minutes earlier was her source of comfort, turns on the fan and...so it goes on.[10] Impaired shivering and impaired sweating (too much or too little)[11] adds to the internal sense of discomfort. I swear that there is just one day, about mid-April, when the world feels comfy. My go-to strategy overnight is to have a heated bed, often a hot water bottle, and then at the foot of the bed a heavy-duty fan whirring all night!

Because of the faulty wiring when it comes to how those with hEDS perceive their own bodily functions, some with hEDS complain of always feeling too cold, and others complain of always feeling too hot even in the depths of winter, whilst many feel that acute swinging from one state to the other. Frankly it's a mess and many of us give up trying to explain our experience because listening to other people telling us how we could cure our own genetics if only we dressed more sensibly is just exhausting and demoralising.

*I am cold unless it is 25 degrees plus, and once I get really cold I can't warm up no matter how many layers I put on. I find it exhausting being cold all the time.*

Emma

## Heart

It goes without saying that the heart ticks away nicely all by itself without the need for any conscious input from its owner. The sympathetic and parasympathetic divisions of the ANS work antagonistically here, with the sympathetic system preparing the body for fight or flight by releasing norepinephrine, and the parasympathetic system calming things back down again after a stressful adrenaline rush with a nice little dollop of acetylcholine.[12] Those little shots of adrenaline are great in the normal course of events – pushing our heart rate and blood pressure up just enough to help us function during a stressful moment and sharpening our focus so we can deal with what's in front of us. But we also all know those occasions when it all kicks in when we are not required to run away from a wild animal – when we open an exam paper or hear bad news or simply watch a deliciously scary film and something jumps out of the shadows. There is that whoosh and then, as the body realises the danger is past, a lovely coming down as the pulse slows and calm returns.

Those with hEDS are likely to 'jump at their own shadow' or if someone calls their name or the doorbell rings. My mum used to tell me that I obviously had a guilty conscience every time I jumped out of my skin when she tapped me on the shoulder! Now, everyone has this experience – you're deep in thought in the middle of a work project and the world beyond your own skin has disappeared. Someone taps you on the shoulder and you jump. What marks out those with hEDS is the ease with which the response can be triggered, the intensity of the response, the often more prolonged nature of the response and then, as the ANS overcompensates back, the crash accompanied by shaking and dizziness and, often, crying (acetylcholine increases tear production!). Exposure to stimuli doesn't help, familiarity *not* breeding contempt in this jumpy population, and this symptom alone can drive those with hEDS to leave their jobs when they realise that their erratic ANS with its propensity to drive their adrenaline and heart rate up to uncomfortable levels before crashing back down again at the drop of a hat isn't simply going to pipe down with time.

The other side of the rushing heart rate is, of course, bradycardia and, at rest, the parasympathetic division of the ANS can go to its own extreme, dropping the heart rate right down during sleep. As we will see shortly, sleep is a big problem for those with hEDS and one common experience is of being shot out of sleep repeatedly as the sympathetic nervous system realises that the heart rate is really low and comes in like jump leads.[13] During an EDS flare I dread sleep – both as I go off to sleep and in the middle of the night I can fly awake, heart pounding in my chest, gasping for air and then unable to do anything except wait for everything to settle, then to drift back off only to have a repeat performance a little while later. Sometimes the spin-around is just minutes, over and over, and on a few occasions the cycling has been so fast from tachy- to bradycardia and back again that I've called the emergency services because I thought I was going to have a heart attack – thinking rationally when you have had an overdose of adrenaline and your heart is pounding in your ears is not easy.

## Thirst and Hunger

Interoception is the body's awareness of internal states – hunger, thirst, pain, the need to pee and so on. As we have touched on elsewhere, the internal messaging system in the hEDS body tends towards the distorted[14] and, with an ANS busy throwing an almighty spanner in the works, the person with hEDS might find that they either over-feel or under-feel the sensations of some of their internal workings. Those with hEDS often describe feeling confused by their internal messages, and this is certainly true of hunger and thirst. The ANS may well misinterpret even small changes in blood sugar as if the body is going into hypoglycaemia, causing the person to feel trembly, 'hangry' and headachy and then, when they eat, their overdriven system can quickly respond with symptoms of hyperglycaemia such as feeling fatigued, nauseated and with abdominal pain. With an altered interoception, the hEDSer can really feel these changes more than one would expect. Likewise with thirst, from the extremes of not feeling thirst at all to feeling desperately thirsty, finding a settled middle ground can prove elusive.

*I have to remind myself to eat and drink and have sex because I get nearly no signals from my body about it.*

Nadia

## Breathing

As midwives and others involved in preparing women for birth we are used to the humour we raise every time we remind a woman during her antenatal birth prep classes to 'remember to breathe'. We know that, when they are hit by a tsunami of contractions, women can respond by panicking and grab at breaths, hold their breath and hyperventilate. When they consciously manage their breathing they can regain a little physical and emotional equilibrium and be better able to ride the waves of labour and birth.

Women with hEDS have often had a lifetime of erratic breathing patterns[15] and may not even realise that their breathing is a little on the unusual side. At rest, with the parasympathetic part of the ANS in ascendence, the breathing might be remarkably slow, and even periodically absent, and then, as always, the sympathetic division will pop its head up and trigger deep gasps. We are often accused of holding our breath but we really aren't – we are simply not breathing! We always will breathe in again – we're really not broken, just erratic – and we will have good days and bad days, but we can find ourselves thinking about our breathing with that heightened interoception and that can make breathing feel a little awkward. Being asked to breathe to a rhythm can, paradoxically, make us feel quite panicky so the use of meditation as a strategy can take some getting used to.

This disordered breathing can further impact on sleep – as sleep comes over the hEDSer and the 'rest and digest' parasympathetic kicks into nighttime sleep mode, the respiration rate can drop very low. Inevitably there is then a sudden responsive shunt awake with a panicked gasp for air accompanied, of course, with that pounding tachycardia. Even when used to it, it can feel frightening.

*My heart rate is slow one minute and then skyrockets. My blood pressure is always low/normal so keeping on top of it is a constant balancing act. Sometimes I suddenly gasp as I realise I have just forgotten to breathe!*

Kathryn

## Swallowing

Another area affected by the dysregulation of the ANS is swallowing.[16] Of course, our swallow can also be consciously controlled – when eating, for instance – but it continues, regularly every half a minute or so, even when we are not thinking about it. We need to keep swallowing when asleep to stay on top of our nocturnal production of saliva, and when we talk or sing or are simply busy working, that swallow keeps on plodding along.

The swallow in hEDS, as with the other ANS functions, can be a little uncertain. An hEDSer might complain about choking on food, gagging when trying to take tablets or of simply, occasionally, finding themselves unable to initiate a swallow when they choose to. I remember my sister once saying to me, 'Rach, you know those moments when you can't remember how to swallow? Well, apparently, it's not a thing!' *Whaaaat?* I raced home and challenged my long-suffering bloke: 'Do you ever forget how to swallow? So you go to swallow and nothing happens and you have to sit it out until your body remembers what to do?' Cue the blank look! Growing up in an hEDS family, I assumed that this was simply what happened sometimes – the body just can't connect the dots and offer up a swallow when asked. Once triggered, the swallow might not 'flow' correctly, which might be why taking tablets can prove such a trial to some hEDSers and why food sometimes doesn't get down the throat smoothly, leading to gagging and coughing or food 'going down the wrong way'. The simplest of tasks made into a clutter-fest by the dysregulated hEDS ANS.

## Sleep

Fatigue is a huge part of hEDS.[17] This shouldn't come as a surprise when the day is spent trying to stay upright, dealing with pain, and with the body and brain in a constant state of hypervigilance. With a body in such a state of exhaustion, sleep should come easily but, as we have touched on, with the wild fluctuations in the sympathetic–parasympathetic balance, things don't pan out as expected.

The hEDS community often spend frustrating years misdiagnosed with myalgic encephalomyelitis/chronic fatigue syndrome (ME/CFS). But the definition of CFS is that the symptoms cannot be explained by other conditions and that obviously isn't the case with hEDS. Here we know what is going on and strategies can help to alleviate the symptoms even if they cannot eradicate them altogether.

Stripping out the obvious cause of sleep disruption due to pain, we find that in hEDS there is often a problem going off to sleep and then, even if the hEDSer feels they have been knocking out the zeds non-stop all night, they wake up feeling totally unrefreshed. When sleep clinics run studies on the general population they prepare for the 'first night effect' – even when the subject is, to all intents and purposes, asleep, half the brain is in an alerted state, keeping watch all night. It seems as if, for at least a proportion of the hEDS population, the overactive ANS ensures that the body is always in 'first night' mode,[18] with half the brain always ready for action, just in case, and every little noise and disturbance in the environment can give a good old poke to the sympathetic system. Some hEDSers experience those big ANS swings as the body dives too deeply into sleep, only to fly up into a sudden, wide-awake state and then back down again over and over and over...this is exactly the population for whom the morning cup of tea in bed was invented. For some, the need to catch up with sleep can be managed by regular napping whilst others form the 'tired but wired' unable-to-nap community as the body digs ever deeper into reserves to keep watch. All the usual sleep hygiene strategies can offer a little relief but there is a limit, and that limit is called genetics.

## Brain Fog

The term 'brain fog' is rather apt as it describes a rather fuzzy feeling causing a sense of confusion, difficulty in concentration, memory loss and of feeling a little outside oneself. In hEDS, it is thought that the cause may be laid fairly on those super-stretchy veins causing the blood

STRETCHED TO THE LIMITS

to pool in the lower extremities. However, brain fog also appears to be a common feature of POTS so the ANS may be playing its own part.[19] It has been shown that high levels of norepinephrine in the brain can disrupt cognitive function and so there is a suggestion (as yet unproven) that the hyperadrenergic state brought about by raised norepinephrine levels could be what is causing the impaired ability to think straight.[20] Of course, this is a population who are almost permanently knackered so...?

## Anxiety and Panic

Anxiety and panic are extremely common in the hEDS population, with close to 70 per cent being affected.[21] In my own work and experience I can confidently say that I have never met an hEDSer who does not suffer with anxiety and panic, and there is a worryingly high proportion who have been diagnosed and treated for anxiety disorders such as generalised anxiety disorder (GAD), panic disorder and anxiety attacks. Whilst it could be argued that there is no problem with a client who has all the signs and symptoms of having GAD being given that as a diagnosis, what marks out these conditions is that they are all defined as not being caused by medication or any underlying general medical or psychiatric condition. This clearly isn't the case with hEDS and the diagnosing of this population as having an anxiety disorder can greatly delay proper diagnosis and treatment of hEDS along with making them feel unheard and disbelieved.[22]

Furthermore, once they have a psychiatric diagnosis in their medical notes, future medical challenges can incorrectly be seen through that prism. Treatments for anxiety such as benzodiazepines and SSRIs can cause daytime fatigue, interfere with sleep and impair cognitive function – not at all helpful in this population – whilst psychotherapy for clients who don't actually have an anxiety disorder can simply fail to treat the real cause of symptoms and further feed the notion that it is 'all in the head' when, in fact, it is really all in the hEDS![23]

The hEDS body lives its days in an almost constant state of pain and fatigue, whilst at the same time being over-alerted and over-managed by a dysregulated ANS. The more adrenaline is depleted thanks to the over-enthusiastic and swinging response of the ANS, the more, paradoxically, it tries to keep the show on the road by responding to smaller and smaller stimuli.[24] Small changes in the external *and* internal environment, including the menstrual cycle, can trigger profound panic, further depleting reserves and exhausting the poor hEDSer who may well find their work, social and personal relationships begin to suffer.[25]

## Moving On...

So, there we have it – not by any means an exhaustive list of all the symptoms experienced by those with hEDS but certainly an exhausting one! This woman's experience of being in the world is one of injury, pain, fatigue, the malfunctioning of pretty much every one of her bodily systems, anxiety and panic. Far from over-complaining, she might well have learnt, through being ignored, disbelieved or pathologised as neurotic, to under-report her symptoms. She might have struggled to conceive, miscarried multiple times and, now that she is successfully and safely pregnant, her hormonal changes are playing havoc with her autonomic nervous system. This woman has just taken a seat in your antenatal clinic...

# PART II

# EDS and Pregnancy

## CHAPTER 9

# First Trimester of Pregnancy and Implications for Care

## Introduction

As we have discovered, due to the ubiquitous nature of connective tissue and, in particular, collagen, hEDS has the potential to affect the smooth functioning of every part of the human body right down to the way nerve messages are transmitted. In addition, it can even affect the way the workings of the body are perceived. Now, as with other syndromes, not every client you see with hEDS will have all the symptoms outlined in Part I of this book and not every client will experience any of her symptoms to the same degree. Some hEDSers might have a completed bingo card but find that their symptoms do not adversely affect their life such that they feel disabled. Others might be nowhere near a 'full house' but have such severe symptoms that they are unable to live what we might consider to be a normal life. Most with hEDS have got used to managing their array of symptoms and put on a good show of being fine whilst actually carrying a daily load of low-level but insistent pain, and whilst fighting off tiredness against the background rumbling noise of anxiety. With her history of being either disbelieved or sent from pillar to post in search of treatments for each individual symptom rather than being seen holistically, the pregnant woman entering your professional life for the first time may well be feeling defensive – her guard up ready. Having read the previous chapters, your heart may sink the minute you grab the booking notes and fire up your pen, ready to scrawl 'Consultant-led care', but actually, this woman in front of you might well present you with the perfect opportunity to practise 'being with woman' and providing woman-cen-tred care like never before.

*My tummy muscles knew I was pregnant before I did! Overnight, it was like a switch had been flicked and I could no longer tense my transverse and abdominal muscles.*

Hana

## Booking

The good news at the outset is that pregnancy outcomes within the hEDS population appear to be within the realms of normal[1] and whilst, for some, hEDS symptoms worsen during pregnancy, for others, they ease. Your client really needs to hear this straight out of the box. Her life has almost certainly been marred by the feeling that her body cannot be trusted to perform normally in any given situation – heck, she can't even walk through a door without sustaining a bump – and every time she has tried to discover more about hEDS and pregnancy, she has found herself lumped in with the other, more obstetrically worrisome, subtypes such as classic and vascular. Even when she has found articles on hEDS, there is a fair chance that they have been based on single case studies – and, just like the world news, it is the big, scary and rare stories which make it to print, rather than those that say, 'Nothing to see here, move along the bus!'

By the time most hEDSers are ready to meet their midwife, they are convinced that they are destined for an intensive experience of consultant-led care, ending in elective caesarean, and a postnatal life spent dealing with the aftermath of haemorrhage and a ruptured uterus, multiple organ prolapses and permanently collapsed joints. That's if they get as far as term – virtually every hEDSer I have had contact with has been led to assume she will have a premature birth.

It would be easy to imagine, because of this perceived nightmare, that those with hEDS would be breaking down your door begging to be put under the care of a consultant and to have everything that modern medicine can throw at them but let's remember that, more than any of the other EDS subtypes, the hEDS woman is likely to be profoundly anxious and to be very triggered into panic by the slightest provocation.

The idea of a surgical delivery when bruising is easy and healing is slow and, worse yet, that spinal anaesthesia might not work effectively, can be truly frightening. This is a woman who, in all likelihood, is used to her voice being ignored and now she might believe that she is about to lose what little autonomy she ever had.

What I hear time and time again is that these physically and emotionally worn-down women want a little peace and calm, to be listened to and believed, be empowered to make informed choices, and to be trusted to know their own bodies and their own limits.

## Getting All Your Ducks in a Row: Planning Care
### Consultant- or Midwife-Led Care

When a client is asked about her medical history and a syndrome pops up, it is tempting to automatically sign her up for consultant-led care, and if you were to simply run an internet search on EDS you might well come away confirmed in that approach. It should go without saying that if there are any other medical conditions – diabetes, Crohn's disease, lupus, and so on – or, indeed, any co-morbidities to her hEDS such as a diagnosed Chiari malformation, cardiac valve insufficiency or organ prolapse, which would normally necessitate transfer away from midwife-led care, then an early referral to the obstetricians should be on the cards. But, on its own, a diagnosis or suspicion of the hypermobile form of EDS should lead you to explore further and consider all her options, not to automatically sign this woman over for full consultant-led care.[2] If she declares she has a different subtype of EDS such as classic or vascular then, again, consultant care should be recommended. But if this woman has the hypermobile form of EDS she needs a different care pathway.

Sure, at some point along the journey something might emerge that requires either short-term or permanent transfer of care, but at this stage, nothing more than a one-off consultant appointment should be expected. If that. The benefit of an early appointment with the obstetric consultant team would be to review any drug regimes she might be on, explore the extent and impact of any co-morbidities and, if appropriate, run a quick ECG to ensure that any palpitations, random tachycardias and ectopic beats this hEDSer experiences in her life are not a sign of a more significant cardiac issue. It might be that her GP feels happy and competent to do at least some of these checks if the woman would prefer to keep it all as low-key as possible.

A later consultant appointment can provide an opportunity to take a very detailed history about allergies and sensitivities (latex, opiates, etc.) and to make certain that provisions in the unlikely case that a caesarean section is required are put in place, such as care of hypermobile joints during surgery and the potential risk of excessive blood loss and poor healing.

Obstetric consultants need reassurance that this client you are sending in for a discussion has the hypermobile form of the condition and as such, if there are no other concerns aside from the hEDS diagnosis, she should be considered fit for low-risk care in the community. Obstetricians, just like you, can only spend so much time googling syndromes and so they are likely to fall into the same 'seen one type of EDS and you've seen them all' way of thinking, and before you can say, 'Can I just check your blood pressure?' they are putting this woman on a care pathway designed for those with the vascular form of the condition. Yes, they *may* have excessive blood loss at birth and they *may* experience premature birth and they *may* need a caesarean section, but pregnancy outcomes are no worse than the general pregnant population.[3] However, as a result of their dysregulated ANS, they might be more likely than the general pregnant population, and indeed the other forms of EDS, to respond badly to the stress brought about by medicalisation of the environment.

## Consultant Midwives

If your local hospital has a consultant midwife then this client might really appreciate being offered the opportunity to meet with them and voice all their worries, explore the risks and benefits of different birthing settings and care options and, later on, to work on a well-thought-out birth plan to go in her notes. Your client is unlikely to know anything about the role and availability of a consultant midwife so don't wait for her to ask – offer.

## Doulas

In these days of tight budgets and staff shortages, it might be tricky to maintain the sort of one-to-one care from a named midwife throughout pregnancy which would help to keep this woman's adrenaline levels at a more manageable level. A doula can provide a solution to this care vacuum.

There are some doulas who offer antenatal and well as intrapartum support, taking women to appointments with health care professionals and advocating for them, and this might be a good way of ensuring that your hEDS client is able to get steady emotional support when you and your team are not available. A good doula is as supportive of the pregnant woman's partner as of the woman herself and the partners of hEDSers are likely to need lots of reassurance that their woman, if supported gently and thoughtfully, is just as likely to have a good outcome of pregnancy as any other Tom, Dick or Harriet. Like the rest of the world, they see the outside manifestations – the endless bruises and joint injuries, the intestinal and bladder irregularities and the daily downing of painkillers – and can perceive their partner (and their baby) as uniquely vulnerable. They have also stood by her as she has been moved from pillar to post by the medical profession, suffering frequent misdiagnosis and subsequent treatments which have just made matters worse. But they may really not understand the profound impact of the dysregulation of the ANS and how, whilst small triggers might send this woman's finely balanced systems rocking, maintaining an air of calm and normality might just be the best protection they can provide. A skilled doula can support the partner so that they, in turn, can support the woman and thereby increase the chances of this woman having a less invasive, and potentially less complicated, birth.[4]

## Midwife-Led Birth Centre
Well over half of all maternity units in the UK have midwife-led units (MLU). MLUs can be either alongside (AMU) or free-standing (FMU)[5] and, particularly for a primip hEDSer looking for a low-tech journey, if there are no additional concerns over and above her baseline hEDS, there should be no reason not to confidently offer this choice,[6] especially if the unit is within easy reach of her home. The AMU offers the benefits of one-to-one care from a named midwife, more freedom to move, a lower use of pharmaceuticals and, by its very nature, a lower exposure to iatrogenic risks. With its promise of a more quiet, home-like environment within very easy reach of obstetric care if needed, this choice may well prove popular for those with hEDS, particularly the primip.

For the multip, or a primip who finds the noise and bustle of a busy hospital environment too anxiety-provoking, a community-based FMU, whilst potentially having a bit more of a trek to obstetric care if required, may be an easier to reach option than an AMU for a precipitate labourer and feel altogether quieter and more homely.

When discussing the options of either an AMU or FMU it is worth considering the likely skill set and experience of the staff in each. If the integrated unit is staffed by rotational midwives, then the benefits of the regular skill updating that this career pathway provides staff might be offset from a client experience point of view if she is allocated a newly qualified midwife or one who has just spent her last few rotations in obstetric and high-risk areas and so lacks the confidence in using the sort of community-learned skills we will explore in the next part of the book looking at labour and birth. The FMU, on the other hand, might have permanent, non-rotational staff able to offer case-loading midwifery care and who are also very experienced in home birthing, protecting the normal labouring and birthing environment, and have the sort of confidence required when attending an anxious woman who is birthing fast and comes with the smorgasbord of hEDS delights. The benefits of an FMU need to be balanced against the lack of immediate access to obstetric support.

## Home Birth Back-Up Plan

Those with hEDS are more likely to have a precipitate active phase of labour[7] and so it makes good sense, from the outset, to have a back-up plan for a home birth irrespective of whether or not your hEDS client hopes to birth in an obstetric or midwifery-led unit. Knowing that, if she 'goes like the clappers', she and her midwifery team are prepared for birthing at home (that the community team will have details of where she lives and her hEDS needs and birth choices) even if she *plans* to be in hospital can be very reassuring. A reassurance is also needed that, whilst she might start labour before 40 weeks, the likelihood of her being caught out before the 37-week definition of term is no more likely than for any other woman[8] – after all, she has almost certainly been busy googling and now believes that any baby born before the 'due' date is early and, in her mind, early might equate to premmie and premmie means danger! She can rest assured that even if she has her baby at 37 or 38 weeks, it is entirely OK to birth at home if her labour and birth unfolds rapidly but normally. Blindly booking this woman for a hospital birth and then having to fire-fight when she rings into the labour ward pushing and panicking serves no-one and certainly does not put this woman's needs and safety at the centre of your care.[9]

No matter how low-tech a birth this woman (and you) wants for herself, there is still a little over a one in three chance that she needs a caesarean section and just over a 10 per cent chance of her needing the help of ventouse or forceps at birth.[10] Midwives are only too aware that some proportion of these figures are almost certainly due to the 'cascade of intervention'[11] and it is their role as custodians of, and experts in, the normal pregnancy and birthing process to protect that normal as far as possible, whilst being alert to changes away from that. When pregnancy or labour veer off-piste, the aim is to steer the process back on course and, when that is not possible, to transfer to the care of the obstetricians where appropriate. But, in spite of the very best care, some women will require the assistance of an instrumental birthing and that means...drugs! It is more than possible that your client has never had a local anaesthetic in her life and she may be entirely unaware that she is at a significantly increased risk of having a sub-optimal response to an epidural or spinal anaesthesia.[12]

The hEDSer is very likely to be 'POTSy'[13] even if she has never spent nauseating time on a tilt table in order to have her notes stamped with that POTS diagnosis, and she might well be intolerant to a range of drugs due to an underlying MCAD.[14] She will almost certainly suffer from TMJD and, just possibly, have a history of jaw dislocations.[15] So a referral for a discussion with the anaesthetic team would be prudent but, again, this can be arranged further along the pregnancy journey unless there is anything pressing found at booking. The purpose of such an appointment would not be to move the woman to ongoing consultant care but to assess jaw mobility and to discuss appropriate use of medication should, at any point, an epidural, spinal anaesthesia or the use of other medications such as opiates become necessary.

## Physio Referral

With an almost 90 per cent risk of developing pelvic girdle pain (PGP),[16] the hEDS woman in front of you is almost certainly going to need the eyes of a physio on her at some point in the next year or so and, with this woman's potential for developing PGP very much earlier than the non-hEDS population[17] (possibly in the first trimester), and for slow healing, a stitch in time really might save nine! The hEDSer with PGP might find her hips clicking and subluxing slightly with each step when she walks, and be able to feel her symphysis pubis grating painfully. Whilst a pregnancy support belt can help to a degree, careful measuring, fitting and use of the belt or supportive body stocking is essential because, given the super-flexibility of this particular pelvis, care needs to be taken to avoid the belt simply over-compressing the unstable joints and causing even more pain.

Making a referral to the maternity physiotherapy team after symptoms have emerged, especially if there is a waiting list, is counter-productive. Even in the unlikely situation that she never suffers from PGP, this is a woman who struggles with protecting *all* her joints, even when not pregnant, and is in desperate need of a good programme of graded and safe exercises as a preventative measure. Due to the higher risk of injury from exercise, physio-led hydrotherapy, if available, might be a sensible choice. Until that appointment comes through, it is wise to suggest, even in these very early days, that the hEDSer avoids 'loading' her pelvis (and the rest of her wobbly skeleton) by avoiding lifting or carrying heavy bags and by ensuring that she gets as much support with any childcare responsibilities she has as is possible.

## Specific Health Concerns
### Allergies

As we have already seen, the hEDS population is at an increased likelihood of having allergies[18] – food, medications and environmental substances such as cleaning products, latex and perfumes. This woman might be quick to name her penicillin allergy but it might not occur to her to let you know that perfumes and cleaning chemicals affect her, and whilst surgical tapes of any kind may or may not actively cause a rash, they might more easily rip the hEDS skin. So very careful and guided questioning about allergies, sensitivities and skin fragility help ensure there are no nasty surprises further down the line. If she already takes regular antihistamines for allergies and MCADS then the regime needs to be reviewed to ensure pregnancy-safe medications and dosages are prescribed. Skin changes, including an exacerbation of eczema, are common in pregnancy,[19] so advice to take extra care to use soaps, shampoos and laundry products that are hypo-allergenic, non-perfumed and non-biological can help reduce the constant, low-grade irritation of the sensitive skin.

## Anaemia

When offering to take a routine full blood count on your hEDSer, I would strongly suggest you also take iron for serum ferritin levels. The hEDS population, as we saw in Chapter 7, are far more prone to menorrhagia as well as easier to bruise and bleed generally. In addition, their recurrent injuries can lead to more frequent episodes of inflammation, which can increase the risk of anaemia.[20] The haemoglobin (Hb) can remain quite normal even as iron stores deplete until they reach a critical low,[21] and this is a woman who is predisposed to bleed more easily during birth. Anaemia can cause fatigue and depression ante- and postnatally and also have potential impacts on the development of the unborn baby.[22] Knowing in advance if iron stores are depleted to less than 30µg/l in your hEDS client at the start of pregnancy gives you plenty of time to get appropriate treatment in place.[23]

## Blood Pressure

The hEDSer in front of you is very likely to have lower blood pressure than the average woman, most probably due to a combination of increased venous elasticity and a dysregulated ANS.[24] It would be easy to breathe a sigh of relief and simply tell her how marvellous this is for her own and her baby's well-being. But, more importantly, this woman needs advice about keeping her hydration and salt levels stable and to take even greater care than usual when getting up from lying or sitting, and when getting out of the bath or shower. Even this early in pregnancy she may need extra time and support getting up from the examination couch – that head rush can be brutal.

## Dental Care

There is an old wives' saying that women 'gain a child and lose a tooth' for each pregnancy. There is no doubt that dental problems can increase in pregnancy as a result of increased inflammatory response to the microbes causing gingivitis[25] and this is why, in the UK at least, dental care is free to women throughout their pregnancy and for a full year after birth. Bleeding of the gums is more common in hEDS prior to getting pregnant[26] and so your hEDS client really should be advised to be fastidious with her daily oral hygiene and to see her dentist proactively rather than waiting for problems to surface – not an easy sell to a woman who might have experience of having dental work carried out without an effective local anaesthetic.[27]

## Diet

Whilst many hEDSers follow a healthy and varied diet, there are also many who have become more and more restricted in their diet in an attempt to relieve their symptoms, either with or without guidance from a nutritional specialist. Add this to the increased likelihood of gut disturbances and, along with giving the usual advice about taking supplemental vitamin D and folic acid, it might be prudent to request, along with the routine pregnancy bloods, tests to assess calcium and vitamin B levels as these have been shown to be lower in those with hEDS.[28] Alongside encouraging as varied and healthy a diet as possible, there is evidence that vitamin C has an important role to play in building, strengthening and healing collagen,[29] so adding a daily dose of berries, tomatoes and other vitamin C-rich foods might just support this struggling system.

## Epistaxis

Epistaxis (nosebleeds) is more common in pregnancy, with a rate of around 20 per cent compared to 6 per cent in a matched group of non-pregnant women.[30] Epistaxis in the non-pregnant hEDS woman is more common and more prolonged due to the fragility of the blood cell walls[31] so the extra mucosal delicacy of pregnancy can cause a recurrence or increase in nosebleeds.[32] The increased nasal congestion so frequently seen in the whole pregnant population might present more significant challenges to the hEDS woman when it comes to trying to stay comfortable: she needs to take more care when trying to clear her nostrils – a good old blow might produce more than she bargained for.

## Exercise

Those with hEDS need to stay conditioned. The muscles tend to be strong from all that time holding their owner upright, and so the emphasis of exercise in hEDS is on building stability and stamina. Resting or 'taking it easy' even when carrying an injury can quickly lead to further joint instability, increased dysautonomia and increased pain and injury.[33]

Whenever I talk to hEDSers a common theme emerges – we all know that we need to exercise and we all know that our physical and emotional health decline if we don't. But it requires a degree of mental and physical stamina to keep up with our conditioning routine which, frankly, we struggle to dig out a lot of the time because...we're tired and sore and anxious! If, in addition, there is a history of early pregnancy loss, you may well have your work cut out to keep this client moving every day. Walking is safe but, as laxity increases, and with the increased likelihood of PGP, the pregnant hEDSer may find she is more comfortable and less likely to stumble and trip if she uses walking poles to stabilise her hips; it may help if she has her shoe orthotics checked and, if necessary, replaced.

Swimming is also really good exercise in this population but, even more so than in the non-hEDS pregnant woman, your hEDSer may need guidance from a physio to help her manage her lack of proprioception and so avoid injury, particularly in the hips. Rocking up to the local pregnancy aqua-natal class where she may not be properly seen amongst a sea of other women is not the safest choice, whereas a simple plan drawn up by a skilled physio could enable her to get down the pool safely on a regular basis. Likewise, pregnancy Pilates and yoga are fine if done pre-pregnancy, but extra supervision and care in a small group setting is sensible once those pregnancy hormones are whipping around the system causing havoc.

It can be genuinely scary to contemplate getting hot and sweaty if your ANS is all over the shop and you're worried you might have a nasty POTS episode and faint with a baby on board, so gentle reassurance that keeping up with her usual paced activity through the thick and thin of pregnancy is safe and protective against an hEDS flare and can improve the symptoms of POTS[34] is helpful.

For those whose mobility and exercise is more severely impacted by their hEDS, they will almost certainly have a routine of daily stretches to keep muscles toned and reduce pain. These should be maintained throughout pregnancy and be reviewed by the maternity physiotherapist as soon as possible and adjusted accordingly to allow for the pregnancy changes.

As with any pregnant woman, any other exercise that this woman is used to is good to continue for as long as she is comfortable and able to do so, but she should just be that extra bit aware that, as well as her joints being more 'slidey' than usual, her proprioception and balance might be even more out of whack than usual. Once she no longer feels able to undertake her usual weekend parachute jumps, continuing to walk and do daily stretches will keep her gently conditioned.

## Headache and Migraine

As with the general population, the experience of headache and migraine can increase, decrease or stay the same in pregnancy, with symptoms generally improving in the second and third trimesters in line with the more stable hormone levels at those stages.[35] When assessing headache in the hEDS client it should be looked at in conjunction with other aspects of the syndrome, such as POTS, Chiari malformation and cranio-cervical instability. Input from the maternity physio team can help where headache worsens due to increased mobility in the neck and spine, whilst managing hydration and salt intake will be useful for the POTSy woman. Migraine medication should be reviewed whilst, again, taking care to look at the EDS-ness of this client rather than solely looking through the prism of headache – a neck brace might be more use than a change to migraine medication.

## Hearing Changes and Tinnitus

Hormonal changes affecting blood volume and blood pressure can impact the functioning of the inner ear and trigger or exacerbate tinnitus.[36] You'll remember from Chapter 5 on the ears, nose and throat that the hEDS inner ear can be particularly bothersome due to increased movement of the bones and the altered nerve conduction. So, for those with hEDS who suffer with tinnitus, the increased laxity brought about by pregnancy can make for noisy days and nights. Tinnitus can be extremely emotionally draining and treating tinnitus in the client with hEDS can be very frustrating – white noise can simply cause 'competitive tinnitus' and there is the additional component of struggling to make quick sense of the spoken word. Many medications, tiredness, anxiety and noisy environments can ramp up the cacophony, further fuelling the exhaustion and worry.

When I talk to hEDSers about their hearing and tinnitus, it has rarely been seen through the lens of their connective tissue issues and they have been steered towards traditional approaches to their symptoms, leaving them feeling defeated. Once they understand the rather different cause of their noisy ears and patchy hearing, the anxiety drops and they can start to work on personalised strategies to ease the racket and clarify the audio messages. A trip to the audiology unit at the local hospital may be useful but the referral letter really does need to highlight this woman's excessive joint laxity so that a more personalised and creative approach using CBT, medication review and, possibly, high-quality hearing aids can be explored. My hearing aids are the first thing I reach for in the morning as they seem to help focus my brain and clarify my hearing, which, in turn, helps to ease the ringing. I have no hearing loss and it was simply good fortune that I saw a brilliant audiologist willing to look at things from a different angle.

## Ligament Pain and Cramps

Along with the early start of PGP symptoms, there is a good chance that, due to the overly stretchy tissues, your hEDS client will be asking you about ligament pain much earlier than you'd normally expect. As the laxity increases with hormonal changes, she might have many new widespread aches and pains, but uterine ligament pain so soon into the pregnancy can be particularly worrying for a new mum when none of her friends are experiencing it so early. Down low in the groin it can, of course, be mixed in with symptoms of early PGP and feel like period cramps, triggering fears of miscarriage.

Remember that there is often heightened interoception[37] and an increased hormonal sensitivity so, to further complicate the sense of imminent loss, there may be an increased ability to feel the normal uterine contractions which continue completely unnoticed in most other women until later on in the pregnancy when they become apparent as Braxton Hicks. I felt Braxton Hicks with each of my four pregnancies from around week 12 and am certainly not alone – a surprising number of hEDSers I have spoken to say they were diagnosed with an 'irritable uterus' because they were experiencing such early 'contractions'. Whether the hEDS uterus is actually contracting more readily than the average womb or if the woman simply feels the muscle fibres doing their regular toning exercises more easily I don't know. There isn't an increased likelihood of premature birth in the hEDS woman, but hormonal sensitivity could maybe make the uterus a little more twitchy? Rather than calling it an 'irritable uterus', which can give the impression of a womb likely to be incited to go into precipitate labour with the slightest nudge, reassure your hEDS woman that (once you've excluded a urine infection, etc.) she really is just feeling the normal healthy working of her uterus more than the average woman and is not about to give birth in the next week or two. Generally the hypersensitive hEDSer will simply get used to feeling squeezes and aches in her lower abdomen and quickly learn that some things, such as a full bladder, being active, being dehydrated and having sex, aggravate it,[38] whilst having a pee and a couple of paracetamol can ease the cramps...for now.

## *Morning Sickness*

Whilst there is no evidenced link between hEDS as a stand-alone diagnosis and an increased risk of morning sickness, for those hEDSers who are very POTSy and sensitive to hormonal fluctuations, there is the evidence it can plague their pregnancies,[39] and that certainly matches my experience of the hEDS community. Already prone to feeling nauseated when getting up too quickly or when hungry or too hot, the early pregnancy whammy of hormonal and vascular changes can be just too much for the POTSy hEDSer. It can start earlier, be more intense and carry on much longer than in the average bod. Treating the symptoms from the POTS angle may prevent worsening at the very least, and might actually lessen the nausea and vomiting. By taking extra care when changing position, eating regular complex carbohydrates and maintaining good hydration day and night, the swinging effects of the dysregulated ANS can be calmed a little. The latter two can be achieved by putting a plate of wholemeal bread and butter and some fruit juice or sugary squash (not the non-added-sugar variety) by the bed overnight so that there is not a prolonged period of fasting leading to a panicky

ANS crash. There are worse things in life than a sneaky midnight feast to stave off throwing up the morning cuppa!

*The first twelve weeks were horrific with sickness to the point where I was bedbound and lost around a stone and a half in weight, and my PGP started early – I had been referred to physio by 11 weeks.*

Alana

## Sleep and Fatigue

The huge hormonal, physiological and emotional changes brought about in the first trimester cause excessive tiredness in a majority of pregnant women.[40] I honestly had no concept of just how profound that fatigue can be before I was pregnant for the first time even though I'd seen enough pregnant women come into my midwifery care. Nothing seemed to help – I could sleep all night and nap every day and still the crashing tiredness completely floored me. Those with hEDS enter pregnancy at a disadvantage when it comes to tiredness – their condition already makes them prone to chronic fatigue to an extent that they might have dragged the CFS diagnosis behind them like a chain before finally discovering the real cause for their semi-permanent state of knackeredness.[41] Now they are pregnant they might well need extra support at work and home to cope with the exhaustion of the early months. Although it can be tricky to get any perceived benefit from extra sleep, resting really is the mainstay of dealing with this first-trimester fatigue. However, as we have seen, maintaining an active lifestyle is essential for pain and movement maintenance in the hEDSer, so this is where pacing and CBT can come into their own as medication-free strategies for both managing fatigue and reducing the anxiety it can cause.[42] For many women, fatigue passes as they enter the second trimester. For the hEDSer, it may ease a bit but not disappear, bringing further worry about how on earth she will cope when the baby is born...

## Varicosities

How we all love a tight stocking! Even without the London Underground map on their legs, the pregnant hEDSer might find support tights help her stay a little more comfortable when up and about as well as keeping her venous return ticking over. This woman doesn't have classic or vascular EDS so she is far less likely to have severe varicosities,[43] but any varicose veins she does have in her legs, anus or vulva will be more prone to getting worse in early pregnancy than other women purely because of the lack of connective tissue support around the veins, and this needs to be taken into consideration when completing the routine risk assessment for thrombosis. There is no doubt that the problem will become more marked as weight increases through the second and third trimester, but early help in the first trimester from a good diet, regular exercise and that delightful pregnancy hosiery might hold back the ravages of the hormonal stretchiness a little longer.

**Note:** When you come to take booking bloods, there is a fair chance that you'll be presented with the bulging veins of your phlebotomy dreams. As you grasp your kit, eyes eager, your client might just, ever-so apologetically say, 'They always struggle to take my blood – just saying!' Put your kit down right now and, with a heavy heart, pack her off to the phlebotomy nurse. Sure, you're thinking, 'It's not your veins that are the issue, you just haven't found the right phlebotomist and, frankly, I'm your girl!' But remember, these glorious trunk roads of veins are likely to collapse the instant your needle touches them and refuse to come back out to play nicely. If your hEDSer does have a great vein which she can guarantee always plays ball, treat it gently, don't go gung-ho with your tourniquet and be careful when taping cotton wool over the injection site – she might prefer to simply hold the wad in place for a while rather than risk irritating or tearing her fragile skin with tape.

\*\*\*

The first trimester – those exhausting, nauseating, scary yet exciting 12 weeks of pregnancy – can seem incredibly long considering that the first month generally swings by without notice. For the woman with hEDS, they can be a foreboding of what is to come as the hormonal and weight changes take grip and her body starts to creak under the strain. Getting a substantial toolbox of strategies in place along with the back-up of a supportive and understanding team at the outset can help mitigate against the approaching storm.

## CHAPTER 10

# Second Trimester of Pregnancy and Implications for Care

## Introduction

Those first dozen weeks pass in a fog of nausea and exhaustion along-side the excitement and expectation that comes with pregnancy. The second three months, from weeks 13 to 28, are, for many women, the time when those rough days give way to a smoother ride and they might feel that 'bloom' they've been promised. For the majority of those living with hEDS, pregnancy makes them feel worse,[1] and, although they may well see their nausea and fatigue ease up, with an increasingly heavier load on an unstable frame and an additional workload putting strain on the extra-stretchy, super-sensitive systems through the body, the reality can really start to bite.

## Considering Consultant Referral

At each step along the antenatal care journey, as with any other woman, concerns might arise necessitating a referral to the obstetric team. Should your hEDS client need such a referral, there is no need to assume that she should automatically remain under their care thereafter just by virtue of her hEDS diagnosis. For this woman in particular, potentially with a history of being misdiagnosed or disbelieved, a visit to the hospital might be more anxiety-provoking than for the average woman and this needs to be accounted for when discussing and making the referral.

## Specific Health Concerns
### Carpal Tunnel Syndrome

The increased vascularity of pregnancy along with increased vasodilation[2] can lead to oedema in the feet and ankles, but also elsewhere in the body, and the hEDSer may be more prone to swelling due to having less tone in her veins and surrounding tissues. In particular she might notice early-onset carpal tunnel symptoms (CTS) which can be remarkably easily triggered[3] – the slight vibrations caused by holding the car steering wheel or pushing a toddler in the pushchair can instigate tingling and pain. Understanding the physiology of how hypermobility in the wrist joints alongside increased tissue fluid can lead to irritation of the median nerve can help the sufferer to manage the use of their hands and reduce the incidence and severity of symptoms. Those hyper-flexible wrists are very prone to poor positioning at night and taking conscious care to use a soft pillow for supporting the hands in a safer position can help to cut out some of the numerous painful wakings caused by totally numb hands (oh, the paradox of pain in a numb hand!).

When they are numb and uncomfortable it is tempting to shake the hands to 'get the blood going' only to exacerbate symptoms by irritating the nerves even more, so showing your client how to hold the hands and wrists still and upright whilst simply wiggling the fingers to get some life back into them is really useful. However, often the only real relief can be gained through wearing shaped splints day and night. Note that using crutches for PGP might well exacerbate the CTS and using wrist splints can make using crutches trickier. There is no easy solution here except for respectful understanding that life through an hEDS-affected pregnancy can be very tough and rob the most cheery soul of humour and resilience.

### Fatigue

Some hEDSers will, indeed, bloom during their second trimester. Most stagger through getting sick of the sound of their own voice moaning about how hard it is. Hormonal changes affect the way women sleep at night with the rising progesterone levels leading to increased sleepiness, whilst oxytocin causes fragmentation of overnight sleep.[4] In addition there is the heartburn and the restless legs and the aching joints, all of which are likely to be of an earlier onset and increased severity when your connective tissue is out of order and you're more sensitive to hormonal changes. We tell women that this is nature's way of getting us ready for sleep-disturbed nights with a newborn, and that might be at least partly true, but sleep still must be had and in our modern society it is rarely possible for the pregnant woman to grab a nap if she is working all day, or running a toddler between nursery and swimming lessons.

Those with hEDS go into their pregnancies with an ongoing sleep deficit, hit pregnancy-related sleep issues earlier and go back to their 'normal' hEDS sleep-affected life afterwards...with a new baby in tow! This woman needs a sleep programme right now – a combination of good, safe pain relief medication, management of reflux, daily paced conditioning exercise and plenty of environmental aids to keep her as comfy as possible in bed. If she is unable to find time in a lunch break for forty winks then she needs to think about how she can adjust her life to ensure she can rest at some point outside of office hours, using pillows and orthotic joint supports to help her rest more comfortably and sleep more deeply. She won't be able to rely on being 'tired but wired' for ever and might simply crash and burn if she doesn't take action.

## Heartburn and Reflux

The nausea and vomiting marking the first trimester can, in the hEDSer, merge seamlessly into heartburn and reflux, the insufficiency of the oesophageal sphincter due to the lax collagen even more compromised thanks to the relaxing effect of pregnancy, causing an increase in symptoms.[5] The reflux can be severe enough to cause ongoing vomiting along with the typical GERD cough as acid bubbles up and irritates the throat. Sipping water, whilst not preventing regurgitation, will, at least, dilute the acid a little and ease some of the burn, but glugging litres in the fashionable 21st-century manner may well simply overfill the stomach and lead to more reflux.

Eating little and often, avoiding spicy and acidic foods, and having the last meal of the day earlier in the evening than usual are all simple dietary strategies worth trying. Lying on the left side at night and when napping can help the stomach contents to stay put due to the anatomy of the stomach, and pillows can be used to raise the head and chest up when the refluxing hEDSer simply has to roll onto her right side so loses the anatomical advantage. She will need to take care to use enough pillows to minimise the risk of simply transferring stress and, therefore, pain to other areas of the body. Over-the-counter as well as prescribed medications for heartburn and reflux can help but need to be chosen carefully as some can cause constipation.

Now, of course, this is all standard midwifery fare – heartburn is, after all, a common complaint in pregnancy – but you can expect to be having this conversation with your hEDS client much earlier than usual and you may find that these strategies become insufficient as pregnancy wears on and the reflux intensifies. If these second-trimester strategies start bottoming out for your hEDSer then consider suggesting the third-trimester tips in the next chapter.

## Mental Health

Women with hEDS are almost universally anxious and prone to panic.[6] A combination of her internal physical struggle due to her altered interoception and her fatigue, pain and dysregulated ANS creates an almost permanent perfect storm and it really takes very little to tip her over the edge into overwhelm. A regular mental health check-in at every midwife or GP appointment, and taking a little time to ensure she is continuing to use all her available mental health management strategies as her pregnancy progresses, is sensible practice. Daily exercise, eating healthily, managing pain and sleep and using meditation and CBT to lessen rumination and panic can often reduce or negate the need for medication in this drug-sensitive population.

> *One of the things I really liked was that I had my health visitor visit me before giving birth so we could talk through some of the issues my EDS could bring in terms of holding baby, my pain, etc. That meant that I could get some strategies in place before I had the C-section.*

Nadia

## Pain

Whether or not the hEDS woman develops significant specific PGP symptoms, she is at a significantly increased risk of generalised pain. Her body was struggling to 'hold it all together' before this pregnancy and, as the weeks go on, the increasing weight and hormonal effects on all her connective tissues can really start to take its toll. Aside from every limb, joint and muscle being prone to aching, she may well find her joints subluxing and, if she is prone to it, dislocating more[7] – I haven't spoken to many hEDSers who have not 'popped a rib' when sneezing, even when not pregnant! If she has not already been referred to an experienced physio then now really is the time to get the support in place with a view to stabilising the body as much as possible with a good conditioning programme. It is worth checking regularly that she is actually keeping up with her programme and supporting her to do so – as obvious as it may seem that, if she wants to reduce her symptoms, she needs to keep up the work, it can be very tough to maintain the enthusiasm for daily swims, walks or stretches when everything aches all the time, sleep eludes you and you manage to pull a ligament or 'pop' a joint whenever you do eventually drag yourself to the Pilates ball!

Increased lumbar lordosis, rolling ankles and kneecaps that refuse to 'track' properly can mean that this woman might well walk at 24 weeks as if she were ready to birth, and also be more unsteady on her feet due to her proprioception failing to keep her grounded and centred. She needs to be advised to have her shoe orthotics checked (and replaced if necessary) and to take extra care on stairs or uneven ground – if she were to fall, she is more likely to sustain an injury and take longer to recover.

If the hEDSer does have significant PGP symptoms, she might well be offered crutches. So now she is hanging her ever-increasing weight from her arms and they are just as hypermobile, so she is quite literally transferring the problem up the line. It might be that crutches are simply a must-have, but the stabilising work has to continue so that they can be used as little as possible, to reduce the risk of sprains, subluxes and dislocations further up this bendy body.

*Hydrotherapy was amazing. The heat of the water and being able to move my joints weightlessly was amazing! It took all the pressure off my hips and pelvis and I could stretch out. Just floating around at the end of the session was the most relaxed my body felt the whole pregnancy.*

Lauren

## Spider Angiomata

There may be no varicose veins but there may well be a sudden proliferation of spider angiomata. These strange little spider veins with a red bump in the middle more commonly appear on the face and neck and are the result of an arteriole becoming distended and then the surrounding capillaries filling up to become visible.[8] The cause of the distension of the arteriole? The failure of the tiny sphincter that normally controls the blood flow into the arteriole...and that sphincter is made up of connective tissue. More common in pregnancy, they can be even more numerous and visible under the thin hEDS skin, and more likely to break and bleed. And boy can they bleed! If they do burst and bleed repeatedly, then, in the short term, cautery can help. In the long term, they tend to disappear once the pregnancy has ended.

## Stretch Marks

Those of us with hEDS are repeatedly told that, thanks to our stretchy genes, we are less likely to develop wrinkles later in life, and so the emergence of stretch marks that can be deep and prolific seems counterintuitive. However, whilst the skin is indeed very stretchy, the collagen fibres are more fragile and prone to fracture. So even though the hEDS skin is super-soft and stretchy, many with hEDS develop stretch marks even before their first pregnancy.[9] Sensitive to circulating hormones and with delicate collagen in their skin, this woman may find her stretch marks multiplying and itching before maximum pregnant bump size has heaved into view and, with her possibly multiple intolerances to laundry products and soaps ramping up the irritation, she might appreciate an appointment with her GP for a prescription for an appropriate soothing cream or ointment to help with the itching.

## Varicosities

As we saw in the previous chapter, although the client with hEDS might well have really visible, plump-looking veins, she does not have the vascular form of EDS and so is not at a greatly increased risk of severe varicosities.[10] However, she is as susceptible as the next woman to have varicose veins and vulval varicosities and, because of the lack of supportive surrounding tissues for her swollen veins, any she does have are more likely to become much worse more quickly. Even if the thrombosis risk assessment was reassuring at booking, as the pregnancy progresses through the second trimester, it is wise to review that assessment and take stock of any varicosities with a view to referral for assessment of prophylactic heparinisation.[11]

## Voice Changes

The relaxing effect of pregnancy hormones can have a noticeable impact on the voice. High levels of progesterone cause the mucus that helps the vocal cords vibrate properly to thicken and reduce in quantity. As a result, the larynx can become dry and the voice deeper and more difficult to maintain. Alongside the increasing upwards pressure from the growing uterus, the ribs flail outwards and the diaphragm has less room for manoeuvre.[12]

The woman with hEDS will very possibly be used to slight changes in her voice production with her monthly cycle, prone as she is to more voice challenges than the average woman,[13] but those changes can be far more profound in pregnancy and, whilst this poses no threat to either her or her baby and so flies under the medical radar, it can be both very alarming to suddenly find your voice becoming husky or deeper, as well as tiring more readily. I remember howling with the upset of discovering myself unable to sing soprano steadily and strongly quite early in my first pregnancy, and no-one could tell me whether this was a permanent change. My reliable stress-relieving weekly singing lesson was lost to me.

Resting the voice makes little difference when it is the circulating hormones making you sing tenor all of a sudden, and a bad tenor at that! But staying hydrated and being reassured that the voice will return to its glorious hEDS elasticity by the time baby is ready to hear you belt out your best rendition of 'Happy Birthday' for the first time can take the sting out of having to sit with the blokes in the local choir!

## Birth Prep

Once the 20-week scan is safely in the bag then it is time to discuss birth preparation classes.[14] This is a client who really should be encouraged to have adequate birth preparation, ideally with a teacher who is familiar with hEDS. The time needed for an hEDSer to explore how her labour and birth might unfold quite differently from the usual may be more than a group setting can provide and so a more personalised, one-to-one offering may be more sensible. This is where a skilled doula can come into their own, ensuring that their client has very robust breathing and relaxation techniques at her fingertips given that she is much more likely to have a fast active labour[15] and be unable to take advantage of pain-relieving medications due to sensitivities, inadequate effect from local anaesthesia and, quite simply, lack of time! As we will see in the next part of the book, on labour and birth, the more the hEDSer is enabled and supported to stay in a low-tech environment, the less exposed she will be to the sort of interventions that might cause more trouble than they prevent. If she is to do this, she must be well prepared and have a good understanding of how her unique body might affect the labour and birth journey, and how she can respond accordingly.

## CHAPTER 11

# Third Trimester of Pregnancy and Implications for Care

## Introduction

The focus for the third trimester when supporting a woman with hEDS is in keeping her as comfortable and mobile as possible and preparing plans for her labour and birth. You will be seeing her more regularly now,[1] and in order to ensure this overly anxious and potentially very sore and tired woman is able to really benefit from the appointments, it might be prudent to protect a little extra time. I know from my many years as a community midwife just how difficult that can be. I also know how much time it can save in the long run.

## Consultant Referral

There is no doubt that pregnancy for the woman with hEDS can be far from an easy ride, but, in the main, the obstacles encountered, rather than being unique and threatening, are simply of an earlier onset and more severe nature than experienced by many non-hEDS clients. With really good support and an ongoing daily conditioning programme, heathy diet and adequate rest, there is just as much reason to assume the pregnancy will end in a normal birthing as the unaffected woman.[2] With her increased likelihood of anxiety, panic, medication sensitivity, decreased response to local anaesthesia, and greater risk of bruising, tissue damage and slow healing, one would have to ask whether maybe everything should be done to keep this woman out of the high-tech labouring environment of a modern obstetric unit and in the hands of an experienced midwife in a quiet and focused midwife-led arena, with fast access to the gadgets and gowns should the labouring journey become more complicated than can be safely managed without their assistance. Where transfer is essential, exposure to interventions should be kept to only the necessary minimum.

Any co-morbidities in your hEDS client should have been picked up at booking and provision made as appropriate but now is the time for a review of current medication regimes ahead of birth and for honing in on the most appropriate place and mode of delivery. A history of hip dysplasia or instability, Chiari malformation, vulval varicosities and malpresentations can sound like a good reason to pack this woman off for a surgical birth but none of these needs an automatic ticket to the theatre.[3] The EDS label simply seems to scare people more than it needs to when prefixed by that little letter 'h'. Those with the classic or vascular forms of EDS are most likely to make up the more concerning stats in the literature. Furthermore, one thing is for sure – a surgical delivery brings a 100 per cent incidence of having an incision and a scar along with bringing other risks – blood loss, bladder damage, drug impacts, and so on. Good midwifery care may well deliver this woman, drug-free, with an intact or minimally torn perineum, normal blood loss and undamaged bladder along with a healthy baby, and we will explore skills to enable this in the next part of this book.

*Compared to hyperemesis gravidarum for the first 20 weeks, the third trimester felt breezy. I think lockdown was in a way a blessing as I didn't have to commute or be anywhere. I could rest as much as I needed and do the exercises that worked for me.*

Emma

## Anaesthetic Referral

Early in this third trimester it is worth reviewing the need for a referral to the anaesthetist. Things to consider are a co-morbidity such as POTS, which might have implications for fluid and blood pressure management during surgery,[4] whether this hEDSer has a reduced effect from local anaesthesia[5] and whether there is a history of TMJD,[6] which might need more careful intubation should it become necessary. Use of adhesive tapes, careful positioning of hypermobile joints and a discussion around any medication sensitivities should be part of any conversation with the anaesthetic and surgical team. Particularly worth noting is the caution needed when using opiates in this population[7] – aside from the fact that they relax smooth muscle and so may be a poor choice of pain medication for those who are quite relaxed enough,[8] they also act on the respiratory centre in the brain, impacting on breathing patterns[9] which, due to the dysregulation of the ANS in hEDS, can already be a little erratic. A surprising number of those I speak to with hEDS describe being overly sensitive to and intolerant of opiates and wish to avoid their use wherever possible.

## Mental Health

I'm not going to beat about the bush here. Those of us with hEDS are a bit of a nightmare to care for. There always seems to be something going wrong with our bodies and, even when there isn't, we're fretting anyway. The sheer unpredictability of living in a body that struggles to know where it is in space, that hurts and that misinterprets its own internal signals keeps the hEDSer in a state of hypervigilance, wrecking the very sleep she needs to soothe and heal her. The hEDS population, as we have seen, is at a hugely increased risk of poor mental health, showing itself primarily in anxiety and panic.[10] Common strategies for dealing with anxiety such as pain medication, regular exercise, healthy eating, protecting sleep, and meditation can become harder and harder to maintain on the hEDS pregnancy journey and we cannot realistically look forward to a speedy recovery after birth.

Antenatal depression is a significant risk factor for subsequent postnatal depression (PND),[11] and this woman will be lugging all the triggers for her current anxiety into motherhood. If a good plan of action to manage this woman's mental health has not been put in place before now, this cannot wait any longer! Antidepressants might well give her a ladder to climb out of her mental pit, but she still has to be able to grab the ladder and climb up it and her hands are in splints and her hips, knees and ankles can no longer support her weight. This is someone who needs a different approach, and the first place to start is sleep.[12]

Sure, she has other kids to care for, and her work to go to, and pain when she lies down but this woman is a grand master at strategising when told that the chips are down and she simply must rest. Whatever it takes – massage, family support, pain medications, a medical sick note...quite simply, if she doesn't get a nap schedule going now then she will literally be in no fit state for dealing with labour and postnatal life. Once she is getting some naps in place she will be better placed to cope with the mayhem that is her hEDS body and mind.

## Deep Vein Thrombosis

Whilst there is no increased risk of deep vein thrombosis (DVT) in the hEDS population,[13] the consequences of hEDS could increase the risk and so it pays to be alerted to the possibility as pregnancy progresses even if the venous thromboembolism assessment (VTE score) at booking was unconcerning. As pain increases, mobility can decrease significantly, weight can increase, and pressure on veins can be significant when there is reduced tone in the surrounding supportive and protective tissues. In addition, hEDSers can have an impaired sense of thirst[14] and whilst some are driven to drink a lot, others tend to run a little dehydrated because they simply don't experience thirst in quite the usual way.

## Gastric Reflux

The heartburn that can start early in the hEDS pregnancy can become brutal as the months wear on. The discomfort can be almost permanent as the oesophageal sphincter laxity is joined by the continual upwards pressure from the growing uterus and its kick-boxing inhabitant. No amount of left-sided lying at night is likely to deal with this level of reflux and it can sometimes be better to suggest the suffering hEDSer simply sits upright overnight. She will need plenty of pillows around her to ensure that her limbs, and her legs in particular, are comfortably supported and resting in a 'normal', slightly flexed, position. A night spent with legs straight out on the mattress can, in the hEDSer, result in prolonged hyper-extension followed by days of significant hip and knee pain, whilst failure to sit with the hips and pelvis straight for any length of time will most likely further increase pelvic girdle pain. Remember that proprioception is often very poor in this community[15] and so, if not vigilant in positioning herself before settling for the night, your client might adopt a position that feels OK but which will really overstretch ligaments, causing damage in the long term without giving the feedback of pain in the short term.

## Pelvic Girdle Pain

As we have seen in the previous chapters, the pregnant woman with hEDS is at a hugely increased risk of early-onset and severe PGP.[16] There is absolutely no promise that this will resolve quickly or fully after birth and some hEDSers continue to have symptoms throughout their life.[17] Using belts and supports to provide stability to the pelvic joints can be at odds with the need to maintain good conditioning of the muscles, tendons and ligaments through using them properly and regularly, which is an essential part of maintaining mobility in the hEDSer – it can be very challenging to square that particular circle. Use of very specific exercises in conjunction with adequate, pregnancy-safe pain relief, careful joint positioning at all times and avoiding lifting and carrying even relatively light objects can help to keep this woman moving. Belts and supports need to be very carefully fitted by a maternity physiotherapist and used judiciously, and the use of crutches needs to be monitored very carefully to ensure they are not simply moving the problem upwards. Bed rest is to be avoided if at all possible – this is not a population that benefits from stopping moving – and, if she is to spend any time off her feet, the hEDSer should be encouraged to enjoy one of her favourite pastimes – fidgeting! If she doesn't already have one, then this is a great time to invest in a birthing ball (often sold as a yoga or Pilates ball) and sit on that when working at a desk as this can help develop core stability whilst gently exercising the pelvic joints and ligaments. Of course, in time, the ball can become an additional birth companion and, later still, an essential bit of baby-soothing kit!

The slipping, clicking and grinding felt when PGP is severe can trigger fear that vaginal birth simply won't be possible without causing damage and further long-term incapacitation, but it is questionable as to whether caesarean birth reduces the likelihood of ongoing PGP[18] and there is the additional concern with hEDS of the potential for slower wound healing and reduced postnatal activity. In order to reassure and protect this woman when preparing for an anticipated vaginal birth (or, indeed, an operative delivery), it can help to measure her pain-free range of movement. With your client sitting comfortably on a chair, ask her to gently open her knees as far as she is able to without pain, then, using a tape measure, record the distance between the knees. This should be the maximum that the knees are ever apart during labour. This is especially important if there is the possibility of using stirrups or if the woman is likely to be unable to feel any pain due to the use of epidural or spinal anaesthesia. Expectation management around the possibility of very slow postnatal PGP resolution and the need to continue with the care and exercise plan (potentially for years) is also helpful – this news, though somewhat disheartening, is unlikely to frighten the hEDSer, who is already used to collecting long-term joint issues like other people collect stamps.

> *Third trimester everything hurt! Everything felt so stretched and my pelvis was about as stable as a chocolate tea pot!*
>
> Rosie

> *PGP to the extreme! Fully reliant on crutches and being unable to move very far made for a very lonely and Netflix-filled third trimester!*
>
> Bekah

## Malpresentations

The lax tissues of the hEDS woman may allow for easier, earlier descent of the foetal head into the pelvis. Just as with the average multiparous woman, the baby of the hEDS primip might engage and disengage quite freely. There is also a better than average chance that it descends and remains in an atypical position. Because so much of the available evidence lumps the various EDS subtypes together, even when they purport to be focusing solely on hEDS, it is difficult to get clarity about non-cephalic presentation at term but, as with any other woman, should the hEDSer present with a baby lying breech, oblique or transverse in the later weeks of the third trimester, an obstetric view should be sought. There is no reason at all why the hEDSer with a breech baby should not be given the opportunity to explore the option of a vaginal breech birth if appropriate, given that the whole body of evidence on breech no longer supports, and acknowledges the risks of, an automatic surgical birth.[19] Bearing in mind the risk of slower healing after surgery associated with hEDS, the potential risk of ineffective spinal anaesthesia and, given the increased stretchiness of the vaginal and perineal tissues, the greater possibility of being able to birth a baby in an atypical position,[20] a genuinely open discussion really should be encouraged and this is where the experience, expertise and client-led skills of a consultant midwife come into their own. There is, of course, the concern around tissue fragility and the possibility of increased perineal damage where there is a diagnosis of hEDS,[21] but there may actually be a decreased risk of anal sphincter damage in this population[22] and really skilled midwife and doula support both during labour and the actual birthing can reduce the risk of any damage. We will explore how best to achieve an intact perineum in Part III of this book.

## Irritable Uterus

The oft-cited risk of cervical incompetence and premature labour that seems to follow hEDSers around like a hungry puppy are simply not very well evidenced.[23] This is one of those areas where cEDS and hEDS appear to have been thoroughly conflated. However, those with hEDS, susceptible as they are to hormonal fluctuations and an increased awareness of their internal workings,[24] can, as we saw in Chapter 9, experience noticeable Braxton Hicks contractions from very early on in pregnancy. Already prone to being hypervigilant and super-anxious, giving this woman the spurious idea that she is likely to birth prematurely and rapidly and that, as such, a close eye should be kept on her cervix through regular assessment of its length, is, at best, questionable.[25] Calm reassurance that she is simply more aware than most of her body's ability to tone the uterus in preparation for an effective labour and birth is a far more realistic and helpful approach. It's worth suggesting she uses CBT to combat her hypervigilance, turning her attention away from the uterine sensations, and to capture and eradicate her anxious thoughts. She may not be aware that a full bladder can trigger Braxton Hicks, as can dehydration, so if she is one of those hEDSers who has a reduced awareness of how full her super-stretchy bladder is and also tends not to know when she is thirsty, this simple sharing of expert knowledge might be just what she needs to reduce the frequency of the contractions.

## Perineal Massage

Is that super-stretchy hEDS skin going to benefit from antenatal perineal massage or is it likely simply to cause bruising? That is the question to which I have no answer as, although there is now a body of evidence pointing to it reducing the incidence of episiotomy and tears (particularly 3rd and 4th degree) as well as pain at three months postnatal in the general population,[26] there is nothing that I can find that looks just at the EDS population. As this is a tribe with a lower incidence of anal sphincter damage during birth[27] then I would be wary of over-enthusiastic promoting of perineal massage and, where an hEDSer does want to do it, would suggest she takes it very easily indeed and does it herself rather than letting her partner do it for her, as she should be better able to gauge when enough stretch is enough!

## Home Birth Prep

As discussed in Chapter 9 when we explored planning the place of birth, even if this woman plans to birth in hospital, provision should always be made for a home birth. Many years ago, when planning a home birth, the maternity pack was left in the pregnant woman's home from about the 36th week of pregnancy. Financial constraints don't make this common practice now but it still seems prudent when the client has hEDS. When faced with the very real possibility of a truly precipitate active stage of labour, even in a primip, it seems foolhardy for a midwife to assess an hEDSer in early, non-active labour and then head off to the maternity unit to grab what she needs, certain that her client has 'a way to go yet'. Cover all bases! Ensure your client has the phone numbers of her preferred birthing unit, any other maternity units and MLUs in her vicinity, a birthing pack somewhere clean and easy to reach, and that her partner has put aside, in a quick-to-find area of the house, a few clean bath towels and has been walked through how to support the woman and 'catch' the baby if midwifery help comes a little too late.

My own husband was a little miffed that I was always so well ahead enough of the game that he was frustrated in his fantasy of the midwife not getting to us and of him being the hero of the hour. I still have the photo from my second birth of the midwife phoning in the birth announcement, red in the face both because she hadn't managed to get her coat off and because she was given a flea in the ear for not having had time to call for a second midwife. Just a few minutes earlier, when she had arrived and I was obviously not 'hard at it', she had told me that I 'had ages yet'!

## Birth Plans

Birth plans first showed up in labour wards in the early 1980s (I started my midwifery training in 1984 and distinctly remember the buzz that greeted them) in response to increasing medicalisation of labour and birth.[28] When individualised and prepared with the support and education of the maternity care team, they can provide an important springboard for discussion as labour unfolds and improve the sense of autonomy and involvement of the pregnant woman in the labouring and birthing journey.[29]

More and more trusts seem to be offering a one-size-fits-all birth plan pro forma in their notes, which seems to me to rather defeat the object and certainly can decrease the sense of true choice.[30] Never is the need for a personalised, well-structured, clear and unambiguous birth plan greater than when it is for a woman with hEDS. Once reassured that, unlike her cEDS cousin, she is really no more likely than the next woman to birth prematurely[31] and, unlike her vEDS cousin, she is no more likely than the average woman to rupture her uterus,[32] and that, thanks to her ability to stretch, her chances of either a caesarean section or an instrumental birth at full dilatation are less than in the general birthing population,[33] the hEDSer can relax a little and begin to plan for her own needs. Use of a 'pick and mix' plan can help her focus on which specific aspects of her labour and birth journey might benefit

STRETCHED TO THE LIMITS

from a more hands-off approach (such as leaving her legs alone) and which would benefit from skilled support (such as active protection of the perineum), and the addition of specific alerts can highlight those unique aspects of hEDS that may alarm care givers who might then interfere too hastily, triggering a cascade of intervention and causing more harm than good.

A good birth plan should be underpinned and supported by robust coping strategies – 'going with the flow' in a precipitate hEDS labour can quickly lead to panic and overwhelm – so encouragement to practise, practise and practise breathing and relaxation for the last couple of months of pregnancy can result in a labour and birth where the woman is more able to communicate her needs more cogently and confidently and so keep herself physically and emotionally safe.

> *My consultant didn't want to do birth plans until 37 weeks, which made me nervous. Baby ended up arriving at dead on 37 weeks and I'd seen the consultant just a few days earlier because I'd been pushy, which was a relief as it meant I'd been cleared to have a midwife-led birth rather than a more medicalised one.*

> Claire

## Birth Plan Specifics

There are a number of topics which, when the birth plan is being drawn up, really require more in-depth discussion:

### Episiotomies, Tears and Suturing

The hEDS skin is, as we have explored numerous times already, really stretchy but also really fragile. It is possible to have an intact perineum with an hEDS birth but the chances are much lower than in the average birthing.[34] Furthermore, performing an episiotomy to avoid excessive tearing might actually cause more problems further down the line as the episiotomy may extend and healing is likely to be slower. There also appears to be an increased risk of prolapse following episiotomy.[35] This is not an argument for never doing an episiotomy, but a stated preference for avoiding one if at all possible through the use of a more hands-on management of the second stage should be considered.

As the head births, there is a natural reflex that women show of drawing their knees together, and this can help open up the pelvis and give more room for the perineum to stretch safely.[36] Requesting that this reflex is left to take place unimpeded might reduce or eliminate perineal trauma as well as helping to avoid excess strain on the pelvic girdle.

Skin in women with hEDS takes longer to heal and perineal wounds are prone to break down as sutures dissolve, so any suturing that is required should, wherever possible, be done with non-absorbable sutures[37] such as black silk. I have lost count of the number of women I have spoken to who have been told that they really don't need 'special' sutures and that it 'isn't possible' to get any ordered in advance, only to suffer, as anticipated, early breakdown of their perineum and slow healing. I have also had the pleasure of speaking to women whose carers have gone that extra mile and secured some black silk sutures in advance and therefore saved them from the considerable pain and upset that a broken perineum can cause at a time when they are trying to get to grips with caring for a newborn. I also speak from the personal experience of having had two experiences with absorbable sutures which broke down and left me with prolonged pain, followed by an altogether happier experience when I was sutured, as requested, with non-absorbable black silk. It is almost impossible to describe just how different the initial and ongoing experiences were. Waiting for the day of labour to think about this is simply too late. This must be thought about in advance when birth planning.

## Management of Third Stage

When discussing the third stage it is important to remind oneself, yet again, that the hEDSer does not have a bleeding disorder or low platelets. She has fragile collagen. This does mean that blood cells and capillaries are more prone to fracture,[38] but not that her uterus is less likely to contract – her prolonged experience of Braxton Hicks contractions and the precipitate nature of her labour should tell us that isn't the problem! When looking at the evidence for increased postpartum haemorrhage (PPH) in the hEDSer, it becomes clear that the major problems are far more likely to be encountered by those with the classic or 'uncertain' subtypes,[39] and whilst one study points to an increased risk of PPH,[40] the cause of the bleeding is not explored although, notably, 64 per cent of the women were given an episiotomy! The finding of increased risk of PPH is not supported by other studies.[41] This is not a reason to be blasé when considering third-stage choices for those with the hypermobility subtype but it should at least be a reason to question the automatic need for a highly managed third stage.

The routine use of active, rather than physiological, management of the third stage of labour (from the birth of the baby to the complete delivery of the placenta and membranes) has many advocates and also many who question its routine implementation, but one thing is clear from the weighty body of evidence – whether active or physiological, good management is essential if haemorrhage is to be avoided. We will explore safe management of the third stage when caring for a woman with hEDS in Chapter 15 of this book, but suffice to say that a good discussion should take place when it comes to birth planning, and the option of a physiological third stage should not be discounted should the hEDSer want to consider that. There is some evidence that, where midwives are experienced in physiological management and where a woman has planned to birth at home, the risks of a postpartum haemorrhage are reduced when the third stage is managed physiologically.[42]

When thinking about planning the use of a uterotonic drug such as Syntocinon® or Syntometrine®, foremost in mind should be that care should be taken during labour to keep the bladder empty, to avoid any cervical, vaginal or perineal trauma during the birth, and that during the delivery of the placenta, any controlled cord traction (CCT) is done with even more care than usual. On this last point, it is worth considering whether, given that CCT doesn't appear to decrease the risk of PPH in an actively managed third stage,[43] the hEDSer, if all is well, should be given the opportunity to push out the placenta even if she has opted for an actively managed third stage. This option might just possibly avoid the potential risk of both bruising of the perineum and also of bleeding if the placenta has not completely separated – there would, in this case, be increased blood loss for any woman, but the increased capillary fragility in the hEDSer could make matters worse. So an open and balanced discussion with the hEDS woman should take place about her third-stage choices and reassurance given that any risk to her of increased blood loss during birth is more likely to be due to tissue trauma than because of a 'floppy womb' and that every step will be taken to ensure her delicate tissues are protected.

## Vitamin K Prophylaxis

Since the 1970s there has been routine use of vitamin K prophylaxis for newborn babies in the UK. Given to reduce the risk of vitamin K deficiency bleeding, its routine use had reduced the rates of the condition to close to zero (when given as an adequate injected dose) until a report in the mid-1980s threw up a possible link between injected vitamin K and an increased risk of childhood leukaemia.[44] Despite this initial finding now being completely disproved, the legacy is that, although the use of injected (IM) vitamin K is recommended,[45] UK trusts now offer women the choice of either IM or oral vitamin K to be given after birth. A minority of women choose to have neither for their baby.

Hypermobile Ehlers-Danlos syndrome is an inherited condition and hEDSers have a 50 per cent chance of having a baby with hEDS: a baby who is more prone to have fragile, easy-to-bruise skin. When the birth plan is being drawn up, your hEDS client needs to know that although, like her, her baby is likely to have just the same level of clotting factors at birth as any other baby, if her baby has hEDS, the risk of increased bruising and bleeding might be higher. It is simply not possible to diagnose hEDS at birth and so she should consider very carefully whether and how she wishes her baby to have vitamin K prophylaxis. If she decides that she would either prefer her baby to have oral vitamin K or none at all, then her birth plan should ideally highlight this and request that she is supplied with an ampule of vitamin K to keep at home after birth in case her little one does show signs of abnormal bleeding or bruising so that a community midwife can visit and administer it quickly rather than her having to travel first to the unit to pick up an ampule. It might also be worth putting a note in the birth plan to flag up the potential for increased bruising and bleeding on the baby's notes in case a second dose is required. I was born, pre-dates, at home at a time when vitamin K prophylaxis was not routine. A couple of days after I was born, I bled. According to my mother, I bled from my nose, ears, vagina and urethra and the midwife, a certain 'Nurse Green', dashed over on her bike and gave me an injection of vitamin K. Hooray for Nurse Green and her frantic pedalling, but my poor mum was scared witless.

## hEDS Alerts

When you are supporting your hEDS client to prepare her birth plan, alongside her other choices and requests, it is worthwhile putting in these 'hEDS Alerts'. I would use a brightly coloured, bold font to contrast with the rest of the plan and include them all, just to be on the safe side.

### Effacement

**hEDS ALERT:** I am at an increased risk of pre-labour SROM. I will call immediately if this happens.

### First Stage of Labour

**hEDS ALERT:** Although my pre-labour may be as long as usual, I am at increased risk of a **PRECIPITATE LABOUR**. Please believe me if I say that I am in very strong labour before you might expect.

**hEDS ALERT:** I may not respond to lignocaine normally. Please take extra care to check that an epidural is effective and be aware that it may need topping up sooner.

**hEDS ALERT:** I have a strong tendency to suddenly drop my BP and increase my heart rate – please take extra care if I need an epidural.

### Second Stage of Labour

**hEDS ALERT:** I am hypermobile. Please take care if using stirrups or when changing my position.

**hEDS ALERT:** My baby is more likely to come down in an unusual position, but I am more likely to be able to birth a baby in an unusual position (including face-to-pubes). Being able to keep mobile may help me. Water is likely to be most helpful for me.

**hEDS ALERT:** I am more likely to tear as my tissues are more fragile. Please help me to birth baby very gently: it might help to allow my knees to be close together rather than open and for my midwife to control the advance and birth of the head (sometimes called a 'slow head birth').

**hEDS ALERT:** I can drop my BP very low and my pulse can be erratic (very low, very high or a mixture). Please alert the anaesthetist if I need surgery.

## Third Stage of Labour

**hEDS ALERT:** I am at an increased risk of heavier, brisk bleeding in third stage (I am not, however, at an increased risk of major PPH). I am happy to have Syntometrine if this happens. Heavier or brisk bleeding is more likely to be due to fragile red blood cells or perineal trauma rather than a failure to either clot or contract.

**hEDS ALERT:** I may not respond normally to lignocaine. Do not suture me until I am completely numb, and please anticipate having to use more lignocaine than normal.

**hEDS ALERT:** I do not heal easily. Absorbable sutures are **NOT REC-OMMENDED** for those with hEDS. Please use **BLACK SILK** if I need sutures. They may need to stay in for longer than is usual.

## After the Birth

**hEDS ALERT:** I cannot hold things comfortably for very long and can damage my joints easily. I have been shown how to hold baby for feeds – this may not look how you expect but please try not to suggest more commonly taught holds as these might cause pain and injury.

\*\*\*

So, we have hobbled through pregnancy in our wonderful support tights and PGP belt, downing antacids like they were going out of fashion and stopping every ten minutes to breathe our way through yet another run of Braxton Hicks and now there is nothing to do except wait for labour to start...

# PART III

# EDS and Labour

## CHAPTER 12

# Latency and First Stage

## Introduction

Your hEDS client is just as likely as the general pregnant population to labour and birth her baby without complications.[1] Moreover, those very aspects of hEDS that so concern obstetricians when faced with an affected woman, such as an increased risk of tearing, bleeding and prolapse, are more likely when this woman is exposed to the very sorts of clinical interventions often brought out to 'manage' those risks, such as episiotomy, and instrumental and surgical deliveries.[2]

So here you have a woman, aching from head to toe, worn out and anxious but who stands every chance, if kept in a gentle, supportive and intervention-free environment, to birth quickly and without complications. Surely she is every midwife's dream? As one of my favourite mentors once said when we raced to a planned home birth only to arrive just a little too late to find a happy couple snuggling their just-born baby, 'Ooh, my favourite type of birth – turn up, have a cup of tea, make sure everyone is fine, and then go home to bed!'

There is no doubt that there could be challenges along the way but, with experienced, skilled and thoughtful care, there is a good chance that those challenges can be overcome and the birthing be safe and satisfying for all involved.

> *Baby born bang on due date. Contractions from 8 p.m., I was happy at home alone (single mum) with my candles and bouncy ball.*
>
> Katie

## Pre-labour

Considering that every last one of us has lived inside a uterus for at least a while and that most of us have made our way into this astonishing world via our mother's vagina, it never ceases to amaze me how little women actually know about their own female reproductive organs and how they work! So it tends to come as a bit of a surprise when their pregnant body begins the process of preparing for labour and birth so far in advance of the 'big day'.

In those last few weeks or so of pregnancy the normally firm cervix beings to soften as the collagen that lends rigidity to the tissues breaks down in a process which is independent of uterine contractions and is more similar to an inflammatory reaction.[3] As the collagen tissue breaks down, so vaginal loss can really increase and be surprisingly watery. For a pregnant woman with hEDS who has been repeatedly warned about premature labour and might well also have been having noticeable Braxton Hicks for some months, this is, understandably, a red flag.

Any diagnostic vaginal examination using a speculum needs to be done very gently, taking care to protect the hips – consider doing the examination with your client on her left side in the same way as some women choose to birth. Choice of any cleaning fluids needs to be cautious to avoid irritation of the sensitive tissues and the actual insertion and opening of the speculum should be done really gently as the vaginal tissues can be delicate at the best of times, and the woman with hEDS is far more likely to suffer from vulvodynia and vestibulodynia[4] as well as being more likely to bruise and bleed.

The outcome of the examination and your own trust guidelines will, of course, inform your next course of action but, as hEDS can make its owner more prone to vaginal infections[5] and mucosal fragility,[6] further invasive checks should be kept to an absolute minimum. In the busy world of midwifery it can sometimes be tricky to keep track of how many examinations have already taken place so it is worthwhile keeping a running total in the margins of the notes to alert any other care givers before they get their gloves on.

## Pre-labour Rupture of Membranes

Although there is a common assumption that, due to the faulty collagen, labour in the hEDSer is likely to be preceded by spontaneous rupture of membranes (SROM), we need to remember that, in spite of women generally talking about 'my waters' and midwives compounding this belief by encouraging the woman to call if 'your waters go', the amniotic sac actually belongs to the baby. So, if the baby does not have hEDS then the hEDSer is no more likely to experience membrane rupture pre-labour than any other pregnant woman, whilst if baby *has* inherited the faulty hEDS genetic, then the membranes may well be more fragile and spontaneously rupture before the onset of either latent or active labour.[7] Of course, this also means that if you are caring for a non-hEDS mother who is pregnant with an hEDS baby, labour might well start at full term but be preceded by an amniotic tsunami! Along with the potentially fragile membranes, potential malpositioning of the head facilitated by the stretchy connective tissues throughout the pelvis can cause pre-labour SROM,[8] but there is no need to do anything that you wouldn't normally do when faced with this situation in any other woman (such as excluding infection, malpresentation and cord prolapse) except to protect those hEDS tissues even more than usual from unnecessary poking.

> *My waters breaking at 37 weeks exactly was my first sign of labour, contractions started within 10 minutes and were immediately full volume and two minutes apart, there was no warm-up! By the time we got to hospital less than one hour later I was already at 5 cm.*

Claire

## Those Term Terms!

Those of us who have worked for any length of time in the world of maternity will be familiar with the women assuming that their estimated date of delivery (EDD) is their 'due date' and that the magic number is 40. We also tend to ask women when they are 'due' and the media, when reporting on the pregnancies of the rich and famous, love to proclaim that they are 'overdue' as soon as the clock strikes midnight at the end of the EDD day. In truth, the length of average human gestation varies between ethnicities,[9] and so the definition of term is 37 to 42 weeks, although some bodies advise the use of early term (37–38+6 weeks), full term (39–40+6 weeks) and late term (41–42 weeks).[10] You know this and I know this but we do have to keep reminding our clients, overwhelmed as they are by 'Google-Garbage' and 'Mum-Myth', that if they birth at 37 week or 41 weeks, they are neither premature nor overdue but quite nicely on time!

For women with hEDS there is the increased likelihood of them labouring during the early-term stage, especially if the head has been engaged for a month,[11] bringing that head down nicely onto a ripening cervix, and the lax ligaments and vaginal tissue allowing even more movement within the pelvis than normal. But that isn't the same as this population being prone to premature labour, which they are not.[12]

## Latency

I find the latent phase of labour fascinating. From an anthropological point of view, this prolonged stage of relatively short and weak contractions, usually accompanied by an adrenalised state of excitement and activity facilitating cervical effacement and descent and rotation of the baby, will have provided ancient women the chance to walk to a place of safety and prepare for the birth. Often followed by a 'rest and be thankful' hiatus, women had the opportunity to eat, rest and recharge before the contractions reasserted themselves in the active phase.

As midwives, we see how stress during this time, such as a trip to hospital, can put the kibosh on proceedings – the body, sensing danger, decides to protect the woman and baby by shutting up shop until the danger has passed and the long 'walk' to the birthing shelter is safe to continue.

No matter how well a woman is prepared during her antenatal care, she is rarely prepared for just how long this phase can be,[13] and most assume that their latent phase is 'true' active labour. No wonder there is often such a mismatch between how long a woman believes her labour to have lasted and what her midwife has written in her notes! Much has been written about the 'cascade of intervention' and its potential for negatively impacting on the course and outcome of what might otherwise have been a straightforward birth,[14] whilst being able to eat normally and having freedom to rest and sleep can make this phase more likely to end in a normal outcome.[15]

The pregnant hEDSer might well believe that the risk of precipitate labour covers latency too, whereas she is just as likely to have a day or two of pre-labour contractions as the average woman. In fact, given that mispositioning of the baby is made more possible due to the lax supporting tissues, she might well find herself at the more extreme end of latency duration and have a spurious pre-labour experience marked by contractions coming and going over two to three days or longer.[16] With the hEDSer's propensity for anxiety and panic, along with a tendency to react strongly to lack of food and drink and to be in a semi-permanent state of joint pain and tiredness, it seems sensible to prepare this woman for the realities of a prolonged latent phase and encourage her to stay in a quiet and supportive, non-medicalised environment for as long as is possible. Eating and drinking normally, keeping the bladder empty, mobilizing gently and also getting plenty of rest will not only help her to prepare her body well for the active phase but might actually help to shorten this latent phase a little.[17]

Whilst opiates such as diamorphine can help women to rest and sleep through this stage, the midwife's positive perception of their helpfulness with the labour experience is not matched by that of the woman, and its use has been under scrutiny for many years.[18] Regular paracetamol along with massage, a heat pack to the back if baby is lying posteriorly (OP), and relaxing in a deep, warm bath can all help to ease an achy hEDS body through the long hours of latency contractions without the need for opiates.

It is tempting to leave the primiparous woman (first-time mum or 'primip') alone in the latent phase and to return to support her once she is establishing in active labour, but it is a trickier decision when caring for the woman with hEDS. Once active labour has begun, things really can go very fast, which can be shocking for everyone and, whereas precipitate labour in a non-hEDS woman might be marked by very powerful, intense and rapid contractions, the hEDS precipitate labour might not present in quite the same way. Whopping great surges are not needed to get the baby through the hEDS pelvis because the path is softer and gives way more easily, and I wonder if this is why so often midwives seem surprised when faced with an imminent birth when the contraction under their experienced hand says, 'Meh – plenty of time yet!' The lovely midwife who I surprised in my second labour had said just that; I had actually replied, 'I think you might be surprised – I think it will be very soon,' and she reassured me that 'these contractions don't mean business yet!'

So it is worth considering how continuous support can be provided for this woman so that she does not find herself alone and frightened. This is where a skilled and experienced doula is worth their weight in gold – able to provide that quiet, supportive presence and spot when her client is sliding into the active phase and now needs constant eyes on her…

> *I had just asked for pethidine, was examined and was at 6 cm so was allowed it. The midwife was taking her gloves off when I said, 'He is here.' She replied, 'Don't be silly, you're only 6 cm.' I insisted he was here so she examined me. She calmly turned to my husband and told him to press the red call button. He arrived before a second midwife could come into the room. My pushing time was recorded as less than one minute.*
>
> Liz

## First Stage

There is, of course, absolutely no guarantee that your hEDS client will go like the clappers and be home before the cat needs feeding – there is simply an increased likelihood. No amount of laxity in the tissues and pelvic joints will rush a baby through a small, android pelvis, and a baby who has managed to get itself into a very quirky position may pose too much of an obstacle to vaginal birthing in even the most h of hEDS women! However, a well-enough-shaped pelvis sat in lovely stretchy tissues is more likely to happily shift around and make way for an acynclitic, persistently posterior (POP) or even persistently transverse (POT) infant than in a less lax woman. There is no evidence for cervical incompetence in the hEDS population;[19] there is simply a lack of resistance in the tissues that normally keep a steadying hand on the labour tiller. The hEDS community is awash with stories of women who felt alone, scared and abandoned as they found themselves suddenly pushing their baby out whilst the staff, despite having been repeatedly informed of the chance of a fast labour, were caught off-guard and unprepared. As I say, I suspect it might be a lack of the typical intensely strong and frequent contractions usually associated with a fast labour that fails to signal the imminent onset of birth.

Even when the hEDS labour is not super-quick, there are still the other aspects of hEDS such as joint pain and instability, POTS and anxiety which necessitate extra care and consideration so, if it hasn't been provided earlier, once the hEDSer is establishing into active labour, she really will benefit from continuous support from someone in addition to her partner.[20]

## Position

Midwifery training focuses on the normality of labour and birth: on how women are beautifully evolved, and their uterus, cervix, pelvis and pelvic floor work together to help their baby descend and rotate steadily. Far from it being 'wrong' for the head to engage in the posterior or transverse position, it is seen as just part of the spectrum of normal and, with good contractions coupled with the resistance of the tissues and the pelvic bones, a long internal rotation will take place and baby will birth in the anterior position – happy days!

When feeling pressured by the clock and surrounded by machinery, it becomes tempting to try and turn the process into a race. Whilst having a labouring woman adjust her position can help to rotate the baby and shorten the labour,[21] and the urge to rotate a baby into the 'optimal' position is understandable when there are concerns about the mother's or baby's condition, when both are coping well with the steadier pace, it seems questionable to try and get the body to do its job faster by repositioning. The last thing the labouring hEDSer needs is to speed things up and, with good care and management at birth, it should be possible to support a baby to turn away from its mum's pubic bone and come to face her backside instead as it makes its grand entrance into the world.

As with the general population, allowing the hEDSer to make the most of any 'rest and be thankful' hiatuses and to find her own position at each stage is more likely to keep her labouring at a pace that feels manageable for her and to protect her joints. Suggestions to try a left lateral or knee–chest position to slow down a speedy journey, or to walk up and down stairs, or hip-hitch if an asynclitic baby is irritating nerves can be useful but, if those positions don't sit comfortably in this hEDS body, then best to leave alone.

**A note for doulas and mums:** Asynclitism describes the baby's head being tilted towards its shoulder as if it's questioning, 'How the heck did I find myself here?' and can be caused by a variety of situations and, in my experience, is often seen in hEDS where a hand has been able to find room inside the pelvis to sit alongside the head and tip it over – then baby really looks like it's asking the question!

Suggest, don't direct would be the most sensible approach. Certainly some positions that are manageable for the average woman can be really hard to maintain for the hEDSer. Sitting upright, unsupported, on a birthing ball is not easy when your spine sags and your proprioception is shot, and even lying on the side poses problems for those with lax hips and ribs. Leaning forward over a sofa or birthing ball with enough pillows to support the arms and shoulders can allow the legs to stay safely together whilst freeing up the back for massage when that POP baby is pressing back hard, and being able to fidget and shift about frequently is safer for hypermobile joints than maintaining any one position for any length of time.

Having free movement limited is rough for any labouring woman and there is no supportive evidence for routine continuous CTG monitoring in the low-risk woman[22] so, unless medically indicated, monitoring should be intermittent and of a type that allows the woman to stay in her chosen position.[23] Most units have waterproof hand-held Doppler and, if you don't have one already in your midwife's kit, the pinard that has a full-length stethoscope attached is fabulous for being able to 'listen in', whatever position your client is currently in, without having to contort yourself. Of course, if you also have hEDS then contortions won't pose a problem!

**Note:** Particularly for the POTSy woman, any change of position needs to be done carefully to avoid head-rush, nausea and tachycardia.

## Food and Drink

Many women feel the urge to 'carb-up' in the run-up to labour. Being encouraged to keep the body fuelled for work appears to shorten latency and, whilst it may or may not impact on whether or not the labour ends in a caesarean section, it does impact on the woman's sense of well-being and ability to cope.[24] For the POTSy hEDSer the thought of not being able to eat and drink as she wishes can be very worrying. The sensation of being 'hypo' and feeling shaky and weak can kick in when the blood sugar is actually perfectly normal, such is the dysregulation of the ANS (read all about this in Chapter 8). A regular intake of fluids and salts will help to keep her free from dizzying head-rush and nausea whilst managing her pulse and blood pressure within a more normal range.

There is a little research evidence on management of labour and birth in women affected by POTS but, frustratingly if rather wearyingly and unsurprisingly, it is all on the subject of drugs and mode of delivery and none at all on the best ways to keep the woman comfortable. Once active labour is in full swing, sips of a sports drink and tiny nibbles of brown bread with salted butter, or spread with a sprinkle of salt, in between contractions will help to keep hydration ticking over in a POTS-friendly way when munching down on a packet of ready salted crisps isn't fancied. Rather than asking if she wants anything to eat or drink, it is always better with the in-the-zone labouring woman to simply hold out the drinks bottle (not a cup for this proprioception-lacking client) and morsel of food and direct them to 'eat, drink!'

## Bladder Care

We know that, whilst a full bladder can irritate the pregnant uterus and increase the frequency and strength of Braxton Hicks contractions,[25] a full bladder does not appear to impact the course of labour.[26] The main purpose when it comes to bladder care during labour is to avoid postpartum haemorrhage, for which the major cause is uterine atony.[27] The hEDS bladder may well be super-sensitive, in which case keeping it empty is easy and the biggest issue you will face is getting your hEDS woman off the loo long enough to birth her (if she is happy and comfy, leave her there). But some hEDS bladders are super-stretchy and also feel perfectly comfortable as they fill up with enough wee to sail a small ship.[28] Even after birth, when there is often a significant immediate increase in urine output, this bladder-capacity hero may not twig her need to pee. So, to reduce the chances of not only PPH but also of post-natal retention and long-term neuromuscular damage to the bladder,[29] a policy of routine hourly to two-hourly trips to the loo during labour is sensible even if the woman declares no interest in going. Setting an audible alarm on a phone, smartwatch or, if at home, the cooker, can really help when time is flying.

## Skin Care

The fine, fragile hEDS skin really can be very prone to bruising, irritation and tearing. Those with the classic subtype are at even more increased risk but those with hEDS do suffer nonetheless. The softest of tapes left on a little too long can cut into the skin and leave grazes and scabs that last weeks, and cleaning lotions that would seem fairly innocuous to most skins can cause skin flares and itching in the more delicate hEDS skin. The underlying nerves, unprotected by the firm topsoil of robust collagen, are also more easily triggered and so simple things like ripples in sheets can feel aggravating as well as potentially rubbing and irritating the sensitive flesh. You know that princess with her long silky-soft hair and delicate skin who could feel a pea under a stack of mattresses? I'm not the only hEDSer to make the connection…

> *My mum and dad used to read me the story 'The Princess and the Pea' when I was little, and joked (lovingly!) that it was about me – I could feel everything! Even now finding the right mattress and bedding is a nightmare.*

> Lauren

Good midwifery practice involves regular checks of immobile labouring women to prevent pressure sores, ensuring that wet sheets are changed, and that the woman changes position. Immobile or not, the hEDSer needs to shift position regularly and have pads changed as soon as they get wet to prevent chafing. Some hEDSers are so sensitive that anything other than the very softest of sanitary pads will chafe quickly so she should use her own pads wherever possible unless the ones your trust provide are gorgeously knitted from the softest cotton.

Any skin washing is best done with plain water and any tapes needed after taking blood or whatever should be minimally and lightly applied and removed as soon as possible and with real care.[30] Because the damage might not be immediately apparent, it would be wise to document any damage that is visible at the same time as recording the brand and use of tapes and cleaning solutions, along with the location on the body, for future reference and guidance. The same goes for any procedure that might cause bruising – there are obvious times, like venipuncture, when you might expect to cause a bruise but you also need to take real care with seemingly innocuous events – your knuckles against skin during vaginal examinations, for instance, or simply grasping an arm or leg a little strongly might result in a tender bruise cropping up the next day.

## Joint Care

It would be grand to imagine that any labouring woman would be the best person to know what position feels most comfortable for her at any given point, and that the chosen position would not only feel comfy but wouldn't harm her joints. Although I have said earlier that the woman with hEDS should be free to choose her own labouring position, her lack of proprioception means that she might still cause micro-traumas that lead to a short- or long-term increase in pain if left completely to her own devices. She can move her joints to a degree that most women simply cannot. Other women might feel a stretch or burn when stretching to the max whereas the hEDSer might be oblivious. Her limbs stop at their fullest extent but that is sometimes limited by the proximity of the next bone rather than the capacity of the ligament to stretch any further. And so...there is no feedback of stretch or burn.

Although the tissues *can* stretch a heck of a lot, they are more prone to bruising and tearing, and the damage often isn't felt until a day or two later. So whatever position the hEDSer chooses for herself, it can help for an onlooker to simply guide each limb back a little to take the strain off the ligaments, whilst pillows, beanbags and wedges can all be used to support and protect limbs and joints. Those shoulders need to come down out of her ears to prevent nerve entrapment and that tape measure really does need to be brought out every now and then to check the legs are not too far apart, even if they feel fine to their owner. Remember that this woman's PGP is likely to take much longer to settle after birth than the average woman and so she needs all the help she can get to avoid any further strain.

The pelvis needs to open freely to allow easy and safe passage of the baby but, due to the lack of resistance from the surrounding tissues, the vaginal tissues and the pelvic floor, a baby lying POP or POL in an hEDS body may descend with a large presenting diameter and come crashing through fast, knocking the coccyx as it does so, causing potential dislocation and painful bruising postnatally.[31] How much this can be avoided, I'm not sure, but we will explore the possibility of using digital rotation once second stage is well under way in the next chapter.

Careful monitoring of the speed of descent can be done via abdominal auscultation of the baby's heartbeat, noting where the beat is best heard each time. It can also, of course, be done by abdominal palpation but this requires the woman to keep moving out of her preferred position and so could be far too disruptive to the calm of the birthing room. If the baby does seem to be descending fast and in a POP or POT position, being in a forward position such as kneeling and leaning over a beanbag, or even exaggerating that and using the knee–chest position, might help the baby to come down more gently at the same time as skimming past that tailbone, allowing it to move safely back.

My own coccyx got well and truly thumped as my first son ploughed through POT. I felt him drop and the coccyx cracking was so noticeable that, even though I couldn't feel any pain due to the intensity of the contraction, I yelled out. It didn't hurt at that moment but the pain after birth was more intense than I could have been prepared for and the memory is still fresh and vivid. I was upright and walking at the time it happened. Maybe being forward would've helped. Who knows, but it's worth a try when you find yourself supporting an hEDS client through labour and birth.

## Emotional Care

We have explored how anxiety and panic are almost universal in the hEDS population[32] and how, because they are caused by an underlying condition, they can be lifelong. There will be periods of exacerbation and times when the anxiety bubbles a little more quietly in the background, but the dysregulation of the ANS means that it is often not very far from the surface and it won't take much to trigger a panic.

Even when an hEDSer has visited a hospital any number of times, or worked for decades as a midwife, an alarm going off or a door banging unexpectedly can still be enough to make that adrenaline surge and then the wonky ANS roller-coaster sets in as it tries in vain to restabilise. Having been told throughout their adult life that labour presents many dangers to them – prematurity, cervical incompetence, haemorrhage, uterine rupture and prolapse – it is little wonder that most hEDSers I speak at are utterly terrified at the prospect of labour and birth whilst also dreading being in hospital where they have felt so ignored and misunderstood in the past.

Hopefully you have had time during the pregnancy to build a trusting and supportive relationship with your hEDS client and been able to reassure her that, whilst she might labour a little differently, if cared for appropriately she is no more at risk of those scary things than the next woman. Having her carefully drawn-up birth plan stapled to the front of her hand-held and hospital notes will reassure her that her wishes will be seen and that, if any diversion from those needs to be made, an open discussion will take place so that, at every step of the way, she understands what is happening and feels involved in the decision-making process.

Whether the labouring journey unfolds at home, in an MLU or on an obstetric ward, keeping the atmosphere as undisturbed, quiet, gentle and unsurprising as is possible will help this woman to settle and focus on the job in hand. She will have many personal strategies for managing her anxiety – breathing, CBT, distraction...you name it, she will have used them all and found her favourites. Making a note for future birth attenders of what helps can ensure that, when shifts change or you need a meal break, there will be continuity of care even when continuity of carer cannot be maintained.

## Vaginal Examinations

Vaginal examinations (VE) are considered to be a helpful tool in assessing the safe and normal progress of labour and birth, and current guidelines are that they should be offered every four hours in active labour[33] – so from when there are painful contractions *and* progressive dilatation from 4cm onwards: active labour, not latency. In fact, the current NICE guidelines do not recommend routine vaginal examination to confirm a woman is in active labour.[34] A vaginal examination can only give you a snapshot of what is happening at that precise moment and not what was happening in the moments before or what will happen the second you have finished. But few women find them completely comfortable physically or emotionally and, if they are cracking along and struggling to stay focused, the whole palaver, no matter how swiftly carried out, can disrupt the flow of breathing and relaxation, and possibly the progress of labour too. For the hED-Ser there is the additional concern of bruising, and sensitivity to any cleaning fluids, gloves or lubricating gels. Furthermore, the shifting around of the woman who might have just found a position where the speed of her labour is more manageable, coupled with the actual examination itself, might just make a precipitate labour even swifter or a difficult labour even more uncomfortable. Assess the descent of the baby by auscultation of the foetal heart and noting the frequency and relative strength of contractions (remembering that, quite possibly, this body will birth the baby without the need for almighty surges), and listening to the woman herself before deciding whether or not that VE is necessary. What do you plan to do with the information? If the answer is 'nothing different' then maybe consider whether or not the examination is essential right now.

When I talk to hEDSers I'm often surprised by how frequently they remark on how they could tell that labour was powering along and could feel that the birth was not far away. Not in some sixth sense kind of way but in an 'I could feel what was happening inside my body' kind of way. Maybe it is that heightened interoception? It is this sensitivity to the internal workings of the body which, when ignored by birth attenders, can leave the hEDSer, once again, feeling ignored, disbelieved or labelled as neurotic.

If a VE is deemed necessary and your client consents, wherever possible do it without having to move her. She really doesn't have to be moved from her comfy forward kneeling position or even to get out of the warmth and soothingness of the birthing pool. In my own practice, when I have done a VE with a woman in an 'upside down' position, and couldn't quite figure out how to describe the location of the fontanelles and sutures, I have simply drawn what I felt and then rotated the picture! I have also been known to stand still afterwards, eyes shut, moving my head upside down so that I could better visualise what I'd just felt. Surely that's not just me?

Avoid separating her legs more than is essential (can you do the examination with her knees together if she is on her knees or side?), clean her vulva with warm water, lubricate with water or, at the most, K-Y Jelly, use non-latex, powder-free gloves and be very, very gentle to avoid bruising and grazing the tissues. When you have finished and have all the information you need about the well-being of mum and baby, let your client clean and dry herself. She is unlikely to scratch or graze her vulva and perineal area with the cleaning tissue – she is used to how gentle she needs to be.

Having said all of the above, if she labours according to her stereo-type, you won't have time to finish grabbing a pair of gloves before this hEDS woman heaves a groan and you whip around to see the top of the head peeking at you!

## Pain Relief

Considering how many times we see the intense reality that normal labour contractions bring a woman, I am always a little amazed that so many of my midwife friends and colleagues use minimal, if any, pain-re-lieving drugs in their own labours. We are only human after all. But our experience of being 'with woman' teaches us that the ever-intensifying waves of contractions marking our client's experience are physiological and not pathological in nature: that they are not to be feared and can, with good support, be worked with rather than fought against or run away from. Your hEDS woman needs to hear this. Quite simply, she is not a great candidate for drugs in labour and she knows it. Of course, her labour and birth might unfold in such a way that she does need opiates or spinal anaesthesia, but she is more likely either to not have time for drugs or to labour and birth better when in full control of her senses and movement.

Whenever I prepare an hEDSer for labour and birth (and there have been very many), I tell her to approach her labour like a midwife – full of the knowledge that her body has been built and prepared for this journey over hundreds of thousands of years of evolution and that giving birth is a totally normal and manageable part of the female human experience. We hEDSers are a stoic bunch – however much you hear us fret about our latest injury and pain, there is a heck of a lot more that we simply get on with, the anxiety, tiredness and pain simply being our constant running companion. When I chat to pre-labour hEDSers they are far less frightened of contraction pain than of poor management exacerbating their hEDS issues – that they will dislocate a hip or tear and not heal properly. They are more worried about birthing alone due to being so precipitate than they are about not getting a dose of diamorphine, and they are much keener to explore and learn non-pharmaceutical strategies for coping with contractions than of learning about an epidural which, quite simply, may not work so well for them.[35]

### Breathing and Relaxation

Hopefully the woman has been able to access 1-2-1 birth prep classes in later pregnancy which have taught her how to focus on different types of breathing to meet the rigours of a fast and furious experience, and have encouraged her to practise frequently so that her responses are now automatic when a contraction hits.[36] When you are supporting her with her breathing, the ubiquitous deep breathing and advice to 'do what comes naturally' won't cut it with this lady. Deep breathing when sliding rapidly from 6cm to transition in a first labour may well trigger hyperventilation and is unlikely to satisfy the body's need for a more appropriately light and gentle oxygen delivery method, whilst 'what comes naturally' is probably panic! Help her instead to follow the upward rise of the contraction intensity with a similarly responsive style of breathing – moving her breaths up into her chest as the uterus tightens and pushes upwards towards her diaphragm, and then even higher up into the lightest 'throat' breaths before bringing them back down to her chest and then her diaphragm as the contraction eases. This type of breathing in conjunction with conscious relaxation and other non-pharmaceutical strategies can overcome panic by refocusing the mind on the placement and movement of the breath in relation to the upward and downward wave of the contraction, eliminating hyperventilation whilst ensuring the intensely working uterus is getting a steady stream of oxygen to assist it.

## Water Injections

If your hospital trust offers them and this labour calls for it, a sterile 'water epidural' using sterile water injections subcutaneously into the lower back can be remarkably effective, especially where there is a posterior-lying baby causing lower back pain.[37]

## Baths and Pools

Use of a birthing pool or a home bath can give the aching hEDS joints much-welcome relief. There is a bit of an hEDS meme about us really being mermaids who have got uncomfortably stuck on land and, when I am powering up and down the length of my local pool, marvelling yet again how this is the only time I am truly pain- and clumsy-free, I am inclined to agree. The temperature needs to be just right for the hEDS woman, who struggles to thermoregulate and whose head can rush alarmingly as she gets out of the bath, so check as you fill and then continue to check as labour progresses, ensuring that the temperature is adjusted correctly for baby in time for the birth. Apart from the now well-recognised pain-relieving benefits of using water immersion in labour,[38] the freedom to move safely in the water along with the wonderful support it gives to the joints might just help to protect them by resisting their movement a little.

If at home, the hEDSer just needs reminding not to get in the bath if she is alone in the house and not to lock the bathroom door!

## Massage

Who doesn't love a bit of a rub-down with an oily rag? Massage has been used to relieve the pain of labour since ancient times and now we have the evidence to back up its use and benefits.[39] As soothing and pleasurably distracting as it can be in early labour, when cranked up with the right amount of pressure and in the right place, it can really help a woman to get through an intense labour when drugs are not a readily available or appropriate standby.

I was lucky enough to train at a time when epidural use was minimal and so maternity physios taught midwifery students seriously good labour massage techniques. The one that I have used more than any other with the most positive feedback in terms of pain relief is using a firm figure-of-eight massage just over the rhombus of Michaelis using the heel of the hand, and a thick oil to give a little more grip than a thinner one – extra virgin olive oil is good but leave out the garlic and chilli! Done throughout every and the whole of each contraction, the pressure signals reach the brain more quickly than those of pain, thereby 'blotting out' the pain. Keep the rhythm slow and steady, in line with the slower, deeper breaths used at the start and end of each contraction, and ensure the movement is continuous – removing the hand can be quite aggravating to a labouring woman.

For the woman wishing or needing to avoid the use of an epidural, this technique is a must in the midwife's strategy toolbox. Pull it out when caring for an hEDSer and her ability to continue moving freely might assist her baby to dash through more comfortably whilst hopefully rotating into a good position – something which, with its bedrest-imposing necessity, an epidural might impede.[40]

### Aromatherapy

Whether or not your hEDSer wishes to have any form of therapeutic massage, before considering pharmacological forms of pain relief, it is worth offering aromatherapy. It is not really known how it works but it is suggested that it stimulates the limbic system,[41] which deals with memories and emotions. This might explain why frankincense appears particularly useful during transition,[42] the oil being associated with places of sanctuary such as those for prayer and worship, as well as with yoga and meditation. Frankincense therefore speaks deeply to us of easing panic and replacing it with a sense of safety. Used widely now in the labour and birth environment, aromatherapy has been shown to reduce anxiety and pain in labouring women[43] as well as reducing stress amongst staff[44] – surely the only labour pain relief to 'treat' an entire roomful of people in one fell swoop? As always when supporting an hEDSer, you would be wise to tread carefully and check thoroughly for sensitivities to smells if there is a history of MCAD (see Chapter 4) before whipping out your potions.

### Pharmacological Pain Relief

Once in this active phase of labour, opiates are simply not appropriate in a labour that could be very precipitate and, as we have seen, are not the best first-line treatment for the over-sensitive hEDS system.[45] If, for whatever reason, it is thought necessary to give an opiate and the client doesn't, to her knowledge, have a sensitivity to them, consider starting with a small dose and then monitor the effect before giving more. At least that way, if a prolonged labour suddenly gets going in a more standard hEDS fashion, there will be less of the drug to clear from the mother's and baby's systems.

Inhalational analgesia such as Entonox® can be useful for reducing an early pushing urge in transition or when a posterior position is causing rectal pressure but it is important to remember that this hEDSer might have multiple sensitivities, including to medications. A little whiff of gas and air might quickly send her reeling and nauseous.

An epidural has a potential triple-whammy up its sleeve for the hEDSer – it might not work very well, if at all, its lowering effect on the blood pressure might be a bit much for the POTSy client, and the increased hEDS tissue fragility has the potential for increasing the risk of a dural rupture in a population who already have an increased risk for spontaneous CSF leaks.[46]

Extra thought and preparation are needed when considering a spinal anaesthesia or epidural for labour or surgery,[47] and more careful monitoring when sited. Of course, epidurals and spinal blocks reduce mobility significantly at the same time as reducing sensation and so regular but very careful changes of position should be supported to ensure skin doesn't break down and that limbs and joints are protected from injury – just because that hEDS limb can be moved easily in a wide range doesn't mean that it should be!

*I had a planned C-section due to EDS and size of baby at 37+3. The spinal took seven attempts and was not fully effective but we were told another attempt was not really worth it.*

Catt

*I had a placental abruption, meaning I was taken straight to theatre on arrival at the hospital. Unfortunately due to slipped discs a spinal epidural wasn't possible as the point needed wasn't accessible due to disc damage. Therefore I needed a general anaesthetic.*

Emily

## Transition

The slide-zone that is the transition from first stage into the second stage of labour is a strange world to inhabit. Neither truly in one place nor another, hormones surge into the bloodstream which will be very useful for pushing a whole human being out into the universe – adrenaline and testosterone – but just seem to cause mayhem right now. All dressed up with nowhere to go! I love the notion that the hormonally triggered panic and anger, created in spades during this phase, are a highly evolved way of calling our tribe in from their own labours in the field to support and witness the birth of its newest member. Midwives' ears prick up expectantly up and down the corridors when the howls and expletives ring out from the room where 'she's cracking on – won't be long!' – a discernible ripple of excitement warming the busy atmosphere. Such an alien and overwhelming experience for the labouring woman, but bringing that real hope of imminent birth.

When a baby is in a helpful position, transition is often over in just a few contractions, but when there is still some rotation and flexion left to accomplish, it can hang around quite a while. Anyone who has experienced a transition can tell you that time has no real meaning – five minutes or an hour all feel like forever, so keeping a woman's focus right in the present moment with robust breathing strategies and maintaining her energy and hydration by giving little bits of food and fluid in between contractions can help her to keep running towards the finishing line even when she is 'hitting the wall'.

The lax-tissued hEDSer might find that her baby comes down quickly even if it has a very deflexed OP or asynclitic presentation but, then again, it might get caught up, mid-rotation, with that sagittal suture sitting across the ischial spines...deep transverse arrest, said in loud stage whispers to signify the potential horror we have found ourselves in! In the general population you might reasonably wait a while for flexion and rotation to take place at the spines and then, if there is no progress, call for a medical opinion, assuming that if baby doesn't shift no amount of pushing in second stage is likely to birth it without outside help. The baby navigating its way through the hEDS pelvis and vagina and getting stuck at the spines may well not turn but *might* still come through and out, unimpeded as it is by the soft hEDS tissues.

However, there could still be quite a delay in transition and so it is worth trying your midwifery skills to encourage rotation and progress.

There is a popular idea bandied around that the reason human females 'suffer' so much in childbirth is because evolution put the ability to walk upright above the need to birth easily. Of course, the truth is that evolution will always put the continuation of the species above everything else, and the shorter, broader shape of a woman's pelvis compared to her male counterpart is testament to that. Those pesky, pokey-out ischial spines, whilst less prominent than in the male pelvis, are still meant to be there – not an aberration – and are evolved to hold up proceedings a little in order to provide long enough with the right counter-pressure required, like the pelvic floor in second stage, to aid rotation into the very best position for birthing. Time and freedom to move keeps women more comfortable and helps the body do its fabulous work. This very primitive state – almost, it seems to me, like a fugue state – drives the undisturbed labouring woman to adopt positions that are better for this baby in this body in this particular labour, and hEDSers are no different. I would argue that, because of their propensity for increased hormonal sensitivity and interoception, they may just possibly be more likely to adopt helpful positions if supported calmly and confidently.

A squatting position has long been used by women in labour to help the pelvis open up and allow her baby to rotate and descend, and some units have installed squatting bars and birthing stools to make it easier in the institutionalised environment of a modern labour ward for women and their carers to take advantage of the increased pelvic diameters gifted by getting down and grounded.[48] For the hEDSer, no matter how driven she feels to drop down and squat, realistically she is likely to regret it bitterly the following week when her poor hips cry out. So supporting her to get her knees up but kept together by adopting forward-leaning kneeling positions is safer. A supported squat on a low birthing ball or stool is possible, but her hips are still more likely to swing out too far and she might not feel any pain until it's too late. Being leant forward over that ball or stool still allows the pelvis to move as it needs whilst having the added benefit of giving access to a well-oiled hand for a sacral pressure massage. A very low stool (in the home the bottom stair or a toddler step will do) allows one foot up and one grounded, which can wiggle an acynclitic baby out of its quirky pose. Stair walking can have a similar effect and is a popular 'trick' with community midwives attending women at home who are wanting to nudge a baby out of its acynclitic position – an upstairs loo and a downstairs labour nest is ideal as you can kill two birds with one stone at every loo break.

When I found myself in deeply deep transverse arrest with my first son I was fortunate enough to have a very experienced and wise midwife with me. Desperate to overcome the early rectal pressure, I was giving frustrated little heaves and then immediately fretting that I would 'push up' an anterior lip. Coming to my rescue, my wonderful midwife reminded me that a ventouse is sometimes used to gently bring a baby down a little more onto a transitional cervix to help it slide to full dilatation so she said, 'Go for it but keep it really gentle.' And so I did gently push myself slowly but surely, and comfortably, to fully. Nah, he didn't ever rotate out of his OT position but you can't win 'em all and I still pushed him out. In the care of a less experienced midwife, I am certain I would have ended up with a caesarean section. Sometimes it's just as well to stop reading the midwifery book and start reading the labouring woman…

*My labour was slow and I ended up having an emergency C-section. The midwives commented on how I only felt the last half of contractions. I was also very sensitive to the hormone drip.*

Michelle

If a baby isn't showing any signs of rotating despite its mother squatting, doing step aerobics and having a secret 'bit of a push', then a confident midwife might try digital rotation or 'finger forceps'. A rather lost midwifery art, rarely taught or practised now[49] but which has some backing as a technique to shorten the length of the second stage and reduce the likelihood of instrumental or operative delivery,[50] digital rotation should require no analgesia for mum, or strong pressure on the baby's head, and can be done before or after full dilatation.

There are a few techniques described in the literature of which the simplest is to use two fingers to provide the resistance required to aid rotation when the pelvic floor hasn't yet been reached to do its job. During a vaginal examination and with or without the membranes ruptured, the woman is asked to bear down whilst a constant pressure is exerted with the index finger against the lambdoid suture to rotate the baby's head. It can take a few contractions for the baby to rotate and, even when rotation has occurred, it is worth holding your position for a couple more contractions whilst the woman bears down to reduce the risk of reverting to the OP or OT position.[51] Manual rotation can also be learnt and does help induce flexion as well as rotation, but is a more invasive procedure that requires physically grasping the head and aiding rotation using either a few fingers or the whole hand[52] – a rather robust and potentially bruising experience for any woman, and more so for the hEDSer.

Ultimately, a baby labouring through an hEDS mother may or may not get held up at the spines and may or may not rotate and flex into a more regular position but, as the saying goes, 'every little helps' in one way or another, and avoiding the need for ventouse, forceps or caesarean section is more than just a little help. Time, calm support, and flexibility of thought and approach are key to helping this woman get the very best out of her uniquely functioning body.

For any labouring woman, and her carers, transition can be truly challenging. Meeting that challenge involves supporting the woman to ride her adrenaline- and testosterone-fuelled panic whilst making the most of any hold-up to guide her little passenger to get into their best tucked-up position ready to greet the world.

*My official labour time was 40 minutes. I waited longer for a bath afterwards!*

Lauren

## CHAPTER 13

# Second Stage

## Introduction

In what feels like forever and, at the same time, no time at all, transition is over. With a bit of luck and a fair wind, the baby has been afforded enough time and resistance to rotate, flex, straighten up and descend tidily past the ischial spines and is headed ever closer now towards the destination of its mother's magnificently long and bendy cuddling arms.

In times past, no sooner had the last vestiges of the cervix glided over the baby's head than it seemed as if a team of cheerleaders would appear and the labouring woman would be invited by someone on each side of her to 'pop your foot on my hip' whilst a third person gazed earnestly between those legs akimbo and, as the contraction swept in, the rowdy cheering would begin. All that was missing was the glittery skirts and swirling batons that would, at times, have offered a welcome distraction and light relief from the intensity of the directed-pushing palaver! In spite of evidence urging midwives and other carers to stop telling a woman to 'take a deep breath in, hold it, pop your chin on your chest and now push down hard into your bottom as if you're constipated!', remnants of this practice seem to remain.[1] Sure, there is far less Valsalva technique (the breath-holding and pushing against a closed glottis) than previously but there still seem to be directions to 'don't waste that breath – keep it coming, keep it coming...quick breath in and push again!' and to 'push down hard into your bottom'.

Frankly it has always baffled me why, when we talk about the 'pushing reflex', we then feel emboldened to tell a woman what to do. After all, we wouldn't dream of telling her how to sneeze and, if we did, we wouldn't be surprised if everyone ended up in an almighty, mucousy mess! As for pushing into the bottom, surely to goodness when a midwife spends her days with her fingers inside a labouring vagina, she knows that the baby ain't coming out of the woman's bottom. Maybe she is simply too shy to say 'vagina' and means to say to push into her 'front bottom'?

## hEDS-Friendly Pushing

The hEDSer needs, perhaps more than the average woman, to be supported to become deeply connected to what is happening inside her body right now so that she can push only when driven to do so, increasing the pressure when needing to progress and then steadying the pace right down again to give time for the very stretchy but delicate tissues to ease around the head. Those tissues really can yield and stretch so easily but tear in an instant. Remember that, on one hand, the hEDSer is often told that she will retain her youthful looks longer than usual thanks to her über-stretchy skin, whilst also being warned to expect more stretch marks in pregnancy. How can both be true? I like to imagine a thin and very stretchy elastic band – pulled gently it will stretch and stretch and stretch but yank it hard and fast and...it will snap! Likewise with the perineal tissue – it needs to warm and stretch gently with just the right amount of pressure.

The current NICE guidelines suggest that second-stage definitions are split into passive and active and that, for the primip, the active, pushing phase might last up to three hours whilst, for the multiparous woman (second or subsequent birth), the baby would be expected to be born within two hours.[2] That is just active second stage. Where there is a need for rotation, flexion and descent, there may well be a noticeable passive or non-pushing phase. The baby has to have come down below the ischial spines and be in contact with the stretch receptors in the posterior vaginal wall to trigger the Ferguson reflex. It is this reflex that gives women what is often called an uncontrollable urge, but which I prefer to call an irresistible urge, by eliciting an increased release of oxytocin.[3] Oxytocin is often called the 'love hormone' and it can be no accident, surely, that women are flooded with oxytocin at the very time they are about to greet their baby.

If the cervix becomes fully dilated before there is descent below the spines then there may be rectal pressure but without that irresistible urge – a bit like when a sneeze is building but it isn't quite the full ticket yet. Pushing just because the writing on the labour ward board says 'fully dilated' might simply wedge the baby more profoundly onto the spines and cause further delay in rotation and descent at the same time as wearing out the labouring mother and baby. The whole body of evidence looking into directed versus non-directed pushing suggests one almighty shoulder shrug – 'Hmm! Not sure it makes much differ-ence to anything either way'[4] – but, as there is no benefit to directing a woman's efforts, better to give time for those more delicate hEDS tissues to stretch.

As far as using the Valsalva technique is concerned, it is worth remembering that breath-holding whilst pushing lowers the blood pressure – reducing placental flow – and then, as women 'run short' they can reflex-gasp, causing the blood pressure to shoot up again.[5] Your average woman might well feel sick and dizzy. Your POTSy hEDSer may faint. There is also some evidence that using a closed glottis approach may put undue strain on the pelvic floor, causing a decrease in bladder capacity postnatally and an increased descent in the pelvic floor.[6]

Less common but potentially more worrying, the hEDSer is at an increased risk of springing a cerebrospinal leak compared to other women,[7] and this is made more likely by using the Valsalva technique.[8]

As I have said, even when midwives have been convinced to stop directing women to use the Valsalva technique and feel empowered to let the Ferguson reflex kick in and trigger active pushing, they fre-quently still feel the need to coach in other ways. When I challenge colleagues as to why 'all the talk of bottoms' they tell me it's because 'that's how it feels – like you're doing an enormous poo!' Well, as the baby first descends below the spines, there is a bit of backwards travel towards the coccyx, compressing the bowel and causing rectal pressure but, as descent continues, the baby comes forward towards the pubic arch, and continuing to push backwards causes pain as it goes against the natural journey the baby is making.

Head back to the anatomy and physiology books and you will clearly see that the vagina and rectum go in different directions and, in any case, when a woman can feel a baby's head in her vagina, it is a form of mild gaslighting to pretend that she should be feeling it in her backside!

Pregnant women have invariably had sex and, even when they have become pregnant through IVF without ever having had penetrative sex, they still know where their vagina is and have almost certainly 'pushed' a tampon to help remove it. Most of us have a socially instigated need to open our bowels in private – even if we are happy to pee with our partner in the room, having a poo is a different matter. Being expected to do it in front of a stranger can bring on an almighty attack of stage fright – no wonder women hold back!

Reassuring women that, yes, baby is coming down inside the vagina and that is where they can feel the stretching and burning allows us to support them more clearly to use their pushing urges in a more focused and hEDS tissue-friendly way. If the head is advancing too swiftly, the pressure and speed can be reduced in one of a few ways: panting, changing position or pushing in a less effective way. Panting allows the contracting uterus to do all the work but can feel frustrating – like suppressing that full-on sneeze. A position such as knee–chest or forward kneeling over a low birthing stool or stair can help take the foot off the accelerator a little – an upright position can have the opposite effect. Pushing in a less effective way can be really precise in terms of helping progress to speed up and slow down and can be achieved by pushing with varying degrees of noise and blowing. Try it – engage your diaphragm and then either push quietly or with a little or a lot of noise or blowing at the same time as trying to push. The diaphragmatic pressure simply eases by degrees.

Whilst still needing to have the freedom to push only when her body demands, the hEDSer will benefit from this sort of guidance – just following her reflexes may just power her baby out too fast for her tissues. Reassuring and supporting the hEDSer to slow it all down can help her tissues stretch more safely and give baby that precious extra time to rotate.

*I'm thankful every day that my 'pushing' stage was so quick as I honestly felt my pelvis was being snapped in half! My girl is seven soon and I can still remember the pain!*

Katie

## Positions

In order to protect the perineum and pelvic floor from trauma, the ideal is a baby heading down with its head straight, well flexed and with the occiput (back of the head) towards the mother's front. This is the classically defined occipito-anterior presentation but, like all ideals, it can sometimes seem a little elusive. The resistance of the vaginal tissues, the pelvic bones and the pelvic floor all help the baby to achieve nirvana but this level of resistance can be in short supply in the hEDSer and so the cavalry of optimal positioning might be needed. The evidence for using maternal position during pregnancy to change the position of the baby has always been mixed,[9] and the same is true for positioning in labour,[10] but freedom to change position does increase maternal comfort and might possibly aid rotation so is worth a try. The downside is that the literature is so focused on the outcome being speed! So it can be a bit of a balancing act with the hEDSer – wanting to protect her tissues from the potentially bruising and tearing effects of a large presenting diameter whilst also wanting to keep progress on the steadier side of 'going hell for leather'.

*Being in water, my bath at home then the pool at the unit, helped so much in the early stages. My midwife supported me wonderfully during pushing, allowing me to keep hold of the gas and air even when the mouthpiece fell off! Kneeling up on the bed holding the bedhead rails gave me the muscle control and hip joint stability I needed to push.*

Karen

Lying in the right or left Sims position – right Sims for ROP and left Sims for LOP (see Figure 13.1) – which is a sort of exaggerated lateral position,[11] may help rotate a baby who hasn't done so at the ischial spines, but then care should be taken to avoid that urge to rush ahead now that 'baby is in a great position'. Likewise, if a squatting bar, birthing stool or supported squatting position, adapted for those hEDS hips, is used, rotation may be achieved[12] but then progress needs to be kept very gentle.

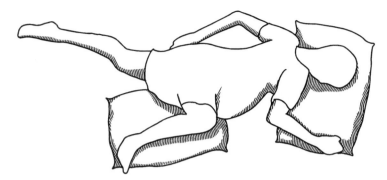

*Figure 13.1 Lying in the Sims position*

## Bladder Care

If there has been a long transition and there is the potential, with a deflexed or acynclitic head, of a longer than average second stage, the bladder can really fill up. Although a full bladder doesn't appear to have much, if any, impact on the course of labour,[13] there are implications for pushing and birthing with one, such as postnatal incontinence.[14] Furthermore, where there is excessive bleeding during third stage, a full bladder impacts on the ability of the uterus to contract fully enough to stem the loss, hence emptying the bladder remains a first-line treatment in the event of PPH. So it makes sense, for the labouring woman's comfort if nothing else, to ensure the bladder has been emptied ahead of active pushing, remembering that some hEDSers simply don't get those full-bladder messages at any time, let alone when there are more important matters at hand.

## Hot Compresses

Oh the joy of a warm compress on the perineum – frankly it seems a waste to only enjoy one during labour! It is one of my happiest memories during my prolonged second stage with OT-boy 35 years ago and its use remains an important midwifery tool for reducing perineal pain all these years on.[15] Although the evidence as to whether or how much a warm flannel held against the perineum whilst pushing reduces tearing,[16] the ability of that compress to reduce pain surely makes it worth its weight in gold.[17] In addition, the woman can hold the compress against her perineum herself, which can give a sense of control and privacy at a time when she might feel vulnerable, a little over-seen and in need of a focus. With a hand over her own perineum the woman can feel the forward journey of the baby – hugely reassuring after all that time, when it is easy to forget what is the purpose of 'all this'.

## Food and Drink

Once a year and always on Mothering Sunday it seems, I get up early to go and help our local Scout group 'man' the water station for the half marathon. The race lasts a few hours, from when those wearing Lycra® shorts and a determined glare rush past, to when those wearing a kangaroo costume and a broad but weary grin jog through. On the 13-mile course there are four drinks stations handing out either water or a sports drink – that is about 300ml every 3 miles and every 30–45 minutes or so depending on your speed. The labouring woman also needs energy and hydration to bring the newest member of her tribe into the world and, for the POTSy amongst us, maintaining a really good fluid and salt balance keeps us upright and clear-headed. A little salt mixed with some honey on a spoon or (my own preference) in a cup of white, sweet tea (how English – 'I drank tea right through each of my labours!') offered in between contractions can help women to feel more positively about their experience[18] and may help them to avoid an energy crash at a vital moment.

## Thermoregulation

Most birthing rooms have heavy-duty fans ready to blast cooling air over the hard-working woman in labour, as well as ruffle the hair of her unsuspecting birth partner. When supporting an hEDSer it is worth just checking in periodically to see if she is still comfy. As we have seen, due to the dysregulation of the ANS (see Chapter 8), the body's natural ability to thermoregulate can be very off-kilter, but this varies from hEDSer to hEDSer, with some always being too hot, others always being too cold and yet others swinging wildly. If you have one of the latter in the birthing room you might need to suggest a combination of a fan *and* thick, woolly socks, or iced drinks *plus* a warm dressing gown.

## Leave Her Legs Alone!

Whenever not encouraging women to push into their bottom as if they're constipated, birth attenders are reminding them to 'open your legs to let your baby out'. We tell them that 'baby needs more room' as we press their knees apart and we mutter to our colleagues over a cup of tea later that 'she kept clamping her knees together on the baby, hanging on to it – she was too scared to let go!' But there really is a reflex urge to draw the knees together, which is as strong, it seems, as the urge of carers to push them apart – I know...I have been on both sides of the birthing space.

The practice of widening the knees to 'make space for the baby' is seen across the world and, when we are trying our hardest to re-empower women to birth more instinctively in line with what their body asks of them, we still seem to believe that, full as they are of primitive, hormonally driven urges, just when evolution should be making birthing easier, it gets this vital bit wrong!

It is time for a big rethink, and the work looking at how instinctively drawing the knees together actually opens the back of the pelvis, making birthing easier and perineal trauma less likely,[19] is as fascinating as it is humbling – why do we still doubt the women in our world?

So put this book down right now, stand up and lean ever so slightly forward with your legs apart. Now take a hand and place the palm over your perineum from behind and feel what happens when you draw your knees together and then take them apart. There you have it! Quite simply, whichever position a woman chooses to be in during second stage, we can confidently leave her legs alone. It is a huge relief with our hEDS woman to be able to throw away the measuring tape, knowing that she will protect her own 'maximum knees apart' measurement if only we can trust her.

## CHAPTER 14

# Birth

## Introduction

When I was training in the early 1980s very few midwives sutured. Even when out at a home birth, if stitches were needed, the GP was called out to do the deed and, when it was suggested that maybe it made sense for midwives to learn to suture, the notion was unceremoniously chucked out. The rationale was two-fold: first, if midwives learnt to suture then there would be less incentive to support a woman to have an intact perineum and, second, GPs were paid to get out of bed and suture – let them earn their money! Within the hospital labour ward the sentiments were the same, and any student midwife needing a doctor to rescue her sorry backside because she had 'allowed' her woman to tear was grilled by the senior midwife in charge – it makes me sweat just to think about it.

Until mass hospitalisation of women for childbirth, midwives were taught to avoid the need for episiotomy and the risk of tears[1] by flexing the foetal head as it began to crown and birth, by 'guarding' the perineum to reduce the stretch, and then by extending the head over the perineum as the face and chin swept upwards away from the anus. Women were also encouraged to pant continuously as crowning became imminent. As they moved into hospitals in the mid-1970s and doctors were more available to suture, episiotomies became commonplace and then, thanks to a backlash by women and pressure groups such as the Association for Improvement in Maternity Services (AIMS) in conjunction with the advent of the Association of Radical Midwives (ARM), tables turned and midwives began relearning perineal protection.

Conversations with colleagues who trained at the same time as me at the start of the backlash and at a variety of hospitals all recount the shame that came with 'allowing' a woman to tear. Where stories differ is in what was taught to overcome the risk of trauma. One colleague was trained to perform an episiotomy on all first-time mothers and on all mothers who had had a previous episiotomy. Needless to say, by the time she completed her training, she had never birthed a woman without doing an episiotomy. By contrast, I trained at a unit with very strong links to ARM and proponents of a more women-centred approach and so I learnt from some wonderfully women-centred midwives how to support a woman to choose her own position, to encourage her to birth the head extremely slowly using gentle breathing or panting, and to use techniques to aid flexion whilst gently watching and 'protecting' the perineum without undue 'fiddling'. An episiotomy, like a tear, was seen as a sure sign that a midwife had not worked hard enough to support a slow and gentle birthing and so, by the time I qualified, I hadn't performed a single episiotomy.

Wherever and however we trained, where those of us who trained decades ago concur is that we simply didn't see third- and fourth-degree tears. There are, of course, other factors to consider apart from much-questioned midwifery practices[2] when it comes to analysing the documented increase in cases of third- and fourth-degree tears (obstetric anal sphincter injuries – OASIS),[3] such as better diagnosis and increased rates of obesity and so, when supporting an hEDSer to birth, we can make the most judicial use of some ancient midwifery skills, updated with some current evidence, to guide the birth of the baby with as little, if any, trauma to mum's perineum as is possible.

Throughout the labour, midwives and other birth supporters work to ensure that, at the same time as keeping mother and baby comfortable, safe and progressing, strategies are used to help the baby move into the optimum position for birth. A baby in the left occipito-anterior (LOA) position at birth is likely to come into the world more easily and do least damage to their mother's tissues, and a well-flexed head coming under the pubic arch is more streamlined and causes less stretching. When we pull a polo neck jumper over our heads, we instinctively tuck our head down and pull the open neck over the crown of our head, down to our ears, and then we start to raise our head as the neck sweeps down over our face. Next time you are a bit chilly and grab that sweater, you will now have a full-on re-birthing experience for which you can thank me!

When it comes to the birthing for a woman with hEDS, it is reassuring to know that the risk of anal sphincter damage may actually be reduced in this population.[4] However, as with the entire second stage, time needs to slow down just enough to enable the tissues to stretch gently and for as much rotation as possible to take place whilst ensuring baby remains in tip-top condition. Slowing things down when the urge to push is huge and the resistance throughout the birth canal and perineal tissues is minimal is no mean feat, but it can be done.

*Despite active labour down as 0 minutes, I managed a slow, controlled delivery whilst standing and not even a graze.*

Erif

## Maternal Position

It seems like an awful oxymoron when I hear midwife colleagues tell me how they believe women should be free to choose their own position for birthing and then quickly follow that up by saying, 'Personally I prefer to use the left lateral!' If your client chooses that for herself, all well and good. Some women are happy and feel able to push on their side but others find it limits their freedom to move and feel involved in the birthing and may also find it more painful.[5] There are other ways to protect the perineum without having to boss a woman into lying in a position you choose for her. Upright positions appear to reduce perineal trauma, but also speed up the journey, which may not be ideal with the hEDSer, particularly if there is still some rotation left to complete. It might be that a forward kneeling position gifts you a little more time, and frees up the hEDS pelvis to accommodate a potentially OP or OT presentation whilst also allowing the knees to stay closer together. A forward kneeling position also appears to have the additional benefits of bringing the lowest risk of OASIS and need for an episiotomy as well as the highest likelihood of an intact perineum compared to all other positions.[6] As with the first stage of labour, when it comes to positions, suggest but don't pressure. Whilst a certain position might afford you a better view of the perineum, right now your hEDS client is going to need phenomenal control of her pushing efforts and she and you need an intensely focused working relationship. Whichever position enables both those elements is likely to be the one that will better protect the super-stretchy, super-fragile tissues.

## Holding Back

As the vertex (back of the head) starts to ease forward, the opening of the vagina begins to open just a fraction – sometimes allowing the vertex to be seen, darkly, deep inside and sometimes not. In the average birthing room, as the next contraction announces itself, a woman may be encouraged to 'really go with your urges now and move the baby round the corner!' The hEDSer on the other hand, just about to swing her baby into sight, needs to be encouraged to ease right off the accelerator – one hefty push might just finish the job at some cost to the perineum, shocking the baby to boot.

Better to encourage a more tentative effort at the start and then gradually ask her to up the power bit by bit than to start all guns blazing and realise, too late, that it was far more than was needed. I made this mistake with my second son – remembering the effort it took to birth my first, OT-son, the second I realised I was fully dilated and had an urge, I launched in with one good heave and felt him fly through and out without any resistance at all. Mutual shock doesn't quite cover the group emotion in the room that evening and I have vivid memories of the suturing that was required as a result of the overly swift birthing.

In a quiet room, the labouring woman in her chosen comfortable position which enables her to really tune in to her body, and with a locked-in connection between her and you (with or without eye contact), now you can watch like a hawk and guide her, second by second, to increase, decrease and hold her efforts during and in between contractions. A held breath along with good use of the diaphragm will give maximum heft, blowing out whilst using gentle diaphragmatic pressure will give a little movement, and panting with no engagement of the diaphragm will allow progress solely as a result of uterine effort. Use a 'Woolworths' approach...pick and mix!

## Perineal Massage

There is evidence that massaging the perineum during active second stage can significantly reduce the likelihood of a severe tear, the need for an episiotomy[7] and postnatal perineal pain.[8] However, it doesn't appear to reduce the risk of first- and second-degree tears and might possibly increase the risk of a spontaneous, albeit non-severe tear.[9] I would suggest that whether or not to do perineal massage is a trickier decision when it comes to supporting a woman with hEDS – those stretchy tissues can bruise so easily, and this is the rationale I was given, as a student, for why midwives shouldn't 'fiddle with the perineum' with a woman under their care – any bruising may put her at increased risk of tearing. However, it is worth considering, especially where baby has not rotated fully and extra room is needed.

Using a water-based lubricant such as K-Y Jelly and wearing latex-free, non-powdered gloves, use your index and middle fingers to massage the perineum with a gentle up-down pressure towards the rectum between the 3 o'clock and 9 o'clock positions.[10] The degree of downward pressure needed should be determined by your client, reducing your pressure if she finds it painful or 'burning'. This can be done both with and in between contractions if and for as long as the woman happily consents. She could, of course, be supported to do it herself – those long hEDS arms and fingers of hers coming in handy, as it were; she is also less likely than you to hurt herself.

## Malpositions

Hopefully there has been enough time and resistance to help the baby rotate into the best position for birth that this woman, with this baby, in this labour can achieve. Aiming for a slower second stage and birth through controlled and gentle pushing should help matters, and if the membranes have remained intact – happy days! If there is an epidural in place then there will almost certainly be a slower pace anyway, but the downside is that, depending on when it was sited, you might be more likely to be seeing a baby come down in a less than optimal position.[11]

If, despite time and positioning during second stage, full rotation has not taken place then, as the head is coming forward now, and starting to stretch the perineum, see if you can support the woman in your care to make use of the unique gutter shape of the muscles of the pelvic floor[12] a little longer by just holding the baby right there against the resistance of the perineum with the most focused of her efforts. There does, of course, need to be just enough of a 'fit' in the pelvis and against the pelvic floor muscles to provide the resistance that enables the final turns to take place. With my midwifery knowledge, I understood the importance of that resistance for enabling stretching, rotation and gentle decompression of the baby's head as it escapes under the symphysis pubis and so, with my fourth – wise after the cannon-firing experience of my second son – I spent a good few minutes consciously using my breath and diaphragm to hold him static on the perineum, which not only helped save my tissues but also gave him time to swivel fully from direct OP to direct OA right at that last moment before crowning – an amazing sensation. It was genuinely hard work to hold him there – the tissues simply don't offer the same resistance to pushes and so that has to be provided by maternal control and support from the birth attendants.

Now that you can see the head you could also try again to provide a 'false' pelvic floor using your fingers as described in Chapter 12 to assist the body to work more optimally and enable rotation before baby begins to emerge.[13]

## Birth of the Head

Crowning can bring the true, sharp 'ouch!' of labour – that intense burn, not dissimilar to the feeling you get when you really stretch the corners of your mouth with your fingers for no good reason. The intense shock causes the woman instinctively to gasp which immediately takes the pressure off and, as the tissues ease a little around the head, the pain subsides and gives way to a sensation of fullness and warmth.

In the past, midwives were taught to use a hand on the occiput at this point and right through the full birth of the head to slow the progress of the head over the perineal tissues (thereby protecting the tissues from sudden stretching), and to aid flexion of the head so that the smallest presenting diameter came through. At the same time, the other hand would be used to 'guard' the perineum and to gently, if necessary, use the fingers and thumb to squeeze together to give a wee bit more slack around the head. This practice came under scrutiny with a number of trials, the best known of which is probably the 'HOOP' study, which was primarily concerned with postnatal pain but which found that a hands-on approach to managing birth increased perineal trauma.[14] However, this study and other similar ones have been more concerned with the practice of squeezing the perineum to give it some slack and not with the slowing down and flexing of the approaching foetal head without touching the perineum – a case of throwing the birthing baby out with the amniotic bath water!

In the average birthing community the vaginal tissues, the pelvic floor muscles and the perineum itself can all be relied upon to temper the force of the uterine and maternal pushes. There is no such get-out-of-jail-free card when supporting the hEDSer and so, if you can see that her efforts, even when held back, are not applying enough of a brake, consider using some manual pressure on the occiput to slow progress and, if needed with a deflexed head, to encourage baby to get their chin down. There should be no need to risk bruising the perineum and this simple intervention may reduce the risk of OASIS in your client.[15] If you feel the perineum does need extra support, that the benefits outweigh the risks and that you feel confident and competent to do so, as you flex the head with one hand, gently use the thumb and index finger of your other hand about 12cm apart, and around 2cm behind the posterior fourchette.[16] By gently pressing your thumb and finger together now, the perineum will slacken ever so slightly around the flexing head. No great force is needed and you need only bring the thumb and finger together by around a centimetre. Although you may indeed increase the risk of bruising and tearing with this strategy, you stand at least some chance of reducing the risk of severe tearing or the need for an episiotomy, which itself can increase the postnatal risk of pelvic prolapse in those with hEDS.[17]

## Still Leave Her Legs Alone!

As we saw in Chapter 13, when a woman is given the freedom to follow her own instincts during birth, she reflexively draws her knees together whilst leaving her ankles apart and that this, far from stopping the baby from coming through, actively gives it more space posteriorly and reduces the risk of OASIS.[18] Even as you support her now to slow the birth of the head right, right down, with, perhaps, the added manual flexion of the baby's head, you should still be able to see the perineum clearly enough to be able to give this focused woman verbal cues and ease the perineum carefully with your fingers. You simply have to shift around however you can to get a good view – I have never had a problem seeing a perineum, no matter what position a woman has chosen for birthing. But then...I am super-bendy!

## Episiotomy

No matter how much you work with a woman to birth gently and to protect her perineum, there are times when the benefit of opting to perform an episiotomy outweighs the risks. A medio-lateral episiotomy at an angle of between 40 and 60 degrees is less likely to cause an anal sphincter injury,[19] and a longer incision which starts around 4.5mm away from the centre of the posterior fourchette is also less likely to extend into the anus. Doing 'just a teeny epis' may not be so sparing for the woman after all. Additional care needs to be taken with the hEDSer to ensure she has adequate pain relief – she may need far more local anaesthetic than you'd normally expect to give and it might wear off more quickly than usual.[20] Waiting until the perineum is distended,[21] there is a contraction and the woman is pushing should thin and numb the perineum enough that whether or not you have been able to get a working local anaesthetic in place won't make too much difference.

## Restitution

There are some midwifery words that are, quite simply, gorgeous. Quickening is one such beauty, and restitution is another. Restitution describes the external rotation of the birthed foetal head as it brings itself back into line with its shoulders as they reach the pelvic floor and rotate in the anterior-posterior position, thereby bringing the anterior shoulder under the pubic arch ready to be born.[22] The time taken for the shoulders to come right down and rotate around can be almost immediately after the birth of the head or it might take some minutes. Whilst the head is out, waiting for the shoulders to descend and rotate, and for the next contraction to kick in, there is no need to rush things along – if those shoulders don't have time to rotate fully, they may simply get stuck or, in that stretchy hEDS body, fly out in the oblique or transverse, causing all the damage you have striven so hard to avoid with the birth of the head. Supporting the hEDSer to continue to 'breathe gently' without any pressure on her to push as this process takes place can help to maintain good perfusion of oxygenated blood to the baby's brain during contractions[23] and for those tissues to gently accommodate the moving body and facilitate the internal rotation.

For the birth partner these minutes seem to stretch forever whilst they watch, feeling helpless, their silent, still, blueish baby just lying there. So many partners have told me how they feared their baby was dead and they couldn't understand why the midwife wasn't doing anything. It doesn't take more than a few seconds to explain and reassure them that all is well, that their child is breathing beautifully through their umbilical cord and that slow and steady really does win the race sometimes. The gentlest of blows on the baby's face – barely more than a whisper of breath – will cause the baby to grimace ever so slightly if proof is needed for the anxious partner that it is OK to let nature do its thing.

## Birth of the Shoulders

Standard midwifery teaching has it that the anterior shoulder should birth first,[24] unless there is a delay due to suspected dystocia, in which case, the posterior shoulder should be assisted to birth first, thereby preventing the anterior shoulder getting impacted behind the pubic bone. However, I have long wondered if the reason it was thought that, left alone, the anterior shoulder would always come first was simply and, quite literally, a point of view. When a woman is lying back and you are watching from above her legs, you can't easily see what the posterior shoulder is up to but, when you can see the entire perineal area easily, many midwives, myself included, would argue that sometimes it is the anterior shoulder, sometimes the posterior one, and sometimes the baby hedges its bets and both come at once.[25] It certainly doesn't seem to affect the perineum much one way or the other.[26]

Standard practice used to be to give downward traction to the anterior shoulder to release it from under the pubic arch, and then, once that had happened, to use upward traction to bring the posterior shoulder up across the perineum. However, that practice has been shown to increase the risk of brachial plexus injury[27] and so, now, if any traction is thought at all necessary as the shoulders birth, it should be as gentle as possible and in the same direction as the baby's spine (axial traction).[28] If given as much time as possible for the tissues to stretch slowly and for the baby to descend and rotate, with gentle support and guidance where necessary, then the hEDSer's baby is no more likely to birth in a quirky position than you'd normally expect.[29]

## The Moment of Birth

The outdated model of that downward traction followed by upward traction to birth the posterior shoulder used to be followed by a smooth ongoing movement of the baby up and over onto the mother's belly – slopped down like a tiny beached whale. The mother's hands, not yet ready to greet her newborn, were often held aloft, startled, as the thrilled attendants encouraged her to 'take your baby!' Anyone who has given birth will remember that moment – still in the weird fugue state of labour, washed about on a sea of hormones, it takes a few seconds to emerge and realise your baby is born. Having that space interrupted and being expected to greet your little one can be too much, too soon. Giving a mother the time to shake out of that moment, as the earth stands still, the umbilical cord pulses and baby has yet to gurgle its first, tentative 'Hello' is a gift. In no time at all, she will come to and be able to discover her baby for herself without it being thrust at her. Then, as she draws her baby in and the oxytocin sweeps over them both like a blanket, the uterus gets back to the work of bringing out the placenta.

## CHAPTER 15

# Third Stage

## Introduction

The third stage – that time between the birth of the baby and the full expulsion of the placenta and membranes – is often considered to be the most dangerous part of the whole labour journey. The care and management we put in place throughout the first and second stages of labour, when we might be more focused on the physical and emotional safety of the baby, the mother and her birth partner, also have implications for the eventual safe delivery of the afterbirth. Avoiding the use of unnecessary interventions, ensuring adequate hydration and nutrition, maintaining good bladder care and supporting the woman to labour in a way that maximises the chances of her baby descending at a steady pace and rotating into an optimal position all help pay forward towards an increased likelihood of a straightforward third stage.

When supporting a woman with hEDS at this stage, it can be easy to let those doubts creep in and to make rushed decisions to intervene. Because birth can more often be truly precipitate when a woman has hEDS it is easy to make the assumption that, as in any other precipitate labour, the uterus has worked too hard, too fast, and that there will, therefore, be an increased likelihood that, once the baby has been safely born, the uterus will decide it's done enough for one day and take a well-earned break whilst someone else worries about the placenta. But that isn't necessarily what has happened in the hEDS body. In this case, the womb hasn't had to work any harder – it's simply met less resistance.

Sure, the hEDSer is a 'bit of a bleeder' but this is due to the fragility of the tissues and capillaries and not that she has a fundamental issues with her ability to clot, and there is little evidence in the hypermobility type of Ehlers-Danlos syndrome that the uterine muscle itself is unable to contract normally – muscle strength is generally good in hEDS.

However, those tissues are more fragile and it is easier to instigate bleeding in the hEDSer than in someone without the condition, so it is little surprise that the literature notes an increased risk of heavy bleeding following a birth in the hEDS population, but the incidence of haemorrhage is more a feature of the classic rather than the hyper-mobile type.[1]

## Active versus Expectant (Physiological) Management

Although we might think that the newly birthed mother would be too consumed with her baby to give two hoots about her afterbirth, very many women do express genuine care about their third stage of labour and how they would like it managed.[2] The debate about active versus expectant third stage has been a hot topic since the Bristol third stage trial hit the midwifery headlines in 1988[3] when its finding that a physiological approach greatly increased the rate of PPH meant that the trial was halted for a while, before being restarted with different inclusion criteria. Since then, the methodology and conclusions of the trial have been thoroughly tested and both upheld and also brought into question.[4]

As things stand currently, whilst the importance of supporting maternal choices is also stressed, a modified active management is recommended whereby a uterotonic drug is given but that cord clamping is delayed for at least one minute (unless contraindicated due to concerns for the immediate health of either mother or baby), and then the placenta is delivered by controlled cord traction (CCT).[5] In spite of these recommendations, it is noticeable that there is a big old question mark over whether or not there is any benefit to CCT in active management,[6] and the risk of PPH appears to be significantly lower when a woman plans to birth at home even if she subsequently births in hospital.[7] The lower risk of PPH in planned home birth may reflect the lack of interference along with the familiarity of the sur-roundings, which seem to make bringing the baby to the breast more straightforward, or the relative experience of the community midwife in managing a third stage expectantly compared to hospital-based staff or both. Whatever the reasons, the debate over best management of third stage is far from finished.

If your hEDS client has asked that her third stage be managed expectantly then, if you would be happy in any other birthing room where there has been a physiological, unconcerning birth to support those wishes, it is not unreasonable to support the hEDSer in hers too. If, however, there have been hiccups along the way which would lead you with any other woman to advise an actively managed third stage then, naturally, the same applies here. It is all about careful moment-by-moment risk assessment and management,[8] and treating your hEDS woman as an individual rather than as her diagnosis.

*I had the injection all three times. The first birth I don't even remember pushing or the midwives pulling it out as I was so out of it. My second and third labour I pushed it out after having the injection. No extensive bleeding or anything.*

Alana

## Postpartum Haemorrhage

One of the popular down-the-pub chat threads amongst midwives following the publication of the Bristol third stage trial was around the definition of postpartum haemorrhage (PPH). After all, the argument went, blood volume increases by an average of 1250ml in pregnancy[9] and that has to be rectified postnatally. Surely, when we manage the third stage expectantly we are simply allowing the body to continue its normal, physiological process to its conclusion, whereas when we intervene to reduce what might actually be a more normal blood loss, we are interfering in that process and any results should be seen in that light?

Maybe, the discussion continued, women who have active management of third stage lose less in the birthing room but then 'make up for it' in those first postnatal weeks by losing more? What about haemoglobin measurements? They may be lower in the first 48 hours after birth in the physiological group but what about further down the line – has the woman recovered her blood loss by six weeks postnatally? In essence, the chat concluded, when it seems that the majority of healthy women are quite able to sustain a loss of up to 1000ml,[10] should we really be setting the first PPH marker at the 500ml used in the Bristol trial?

Hospitals now use the terms 'minor PPH' (500–1000ml) and 'major PPH' (more than 1000ml),[11] but it still seems to me that, alongside our, rather poor, estimations of blood loss, we should be looking at the impact of any loss at all on the mother – even a 450ml loss which might be a walk in the park to one woman could be just too much to the woman already teetering along with a normal Hb but with low iron stores or the hEDSer with a hypervigilant ANS.

You may notice that your hEDS client bleeds briskly as the third stage takes place, but place a hand very gently at the fundus and you should still feel a nicely contracted uterus, especially if her baby is snuggled near or on her breast. The hEDS body seems, to me at least, to be just more enthusiastic than most with their bleeding in third stage rather than more profuse, but it makes sense when supporting a woman with hEDS in her choice for a physiological third stage to have your uterotonic drug of choice very close to hand just in case, particularly where a malposition may have asked more of the uterus in terms of time and effort.

If there is more bleeding and for longer than you feel comfortable with, bear in mind as you set about emptying the bladder and thinking about if and when to instigate your PPH protocol, that if the labour and birth have been essentially straightforward, the loss may well be coming from trauma rather than as a result of uterine atony. Even a small tear in the hEDSer may bleed more easily so do check really carefully for vaginal and perineal trauma whilst also gently assessing the contraction of the womb.

The hEDS body will clot just as nicely as the next body, but knock any injury too soon and you will set the bleeding off again, so this would be a good enough reason to reduce your touching of the perineum and minimise CCT as far as you can as the placenta comes out – as with the labour and birth, use a more gentle approach, giving enough time, whilst keeping everyone safe.

The impact of even a moderate blood loss on a POTSy hEDSer can be more obvious, potentially making assessment of hidden blood loss a little trickier – is this woman pale, nauseous and feeling faint because she has POTS or because she is bleeding more than you can see? Her pulse may not be so helpful an indicator, thanks to the T part of POTS, but her blood pressure may possibly be a little more instructive and a better guide as to the next best steps.

The heat of a birthing pool may be too much at this stage and so it may be wise to support a POTSy hEDSer in exiting the pool as soon as the baby is born rather than wait if she is in the slightest bit wobbly. Good management of food and fluid intake throughout labour should have reduced the risk of a POTS attack at this stage but won't rule it out entirely, so have a second midwife assessing and supporting your queasy client whilst you assess and manage the source of any bleeding.

Accurate assessment of blood loss is notoriously poor in the birthing room[12] and there is currently no evidence that one way of measuring it is better than another.[13] We tend to underestimate at the lower end of loss and overestimate at the higher end but, ultimately, it is the impact on the woman herself of her blood loss that is most relevant, and so a combination of measuring loss as best as possible in the birthing room using our eyes, by collection into a measuring jug and, where possible and appropriate, weighing of bloodstained sheets and pads, close assessment of the well-being of the mother, and adequate testing of haemoglobin and iron stores postnatally should guide our care in this final stage of labour, before we support the new family on the journey into their next chapter.

*I had a C-section: in the surgery the midwife came up and asked my partner if he wanted her to go and take a photo of my placenta. We were all over the place, it was not a question we had the answer to. He said no, then changed to yes and we got the photo, which actually I am quite glad of!*

Lorna

# PART IV

# Postnatal

## CHAPTER 16

# The First Hours

## Introduction

The sheets have been changed, the clock has been read out loud to announce the time of birth (neatly ignoring the fact that the clock in the other room says something different) and now the babe is in arms being thoroughly checked to see if they look more like Mum or their Great Uncle Bob. Right now adrenaline and oxytocin levels are high, bruising and swelling are at their minimum and there is an hEDSer whose perineum, bladder and joints need the very best of your care.

## Mum
### Stitches

It can seem like the cruellest trick of all – after all the sheer physical hard work of labour and birth, just when you want to enjoy those first peach-soft snuggles with your newborn, your poor, bruised perineum is going to get poked around! The majority (around 85 per cent) of women will sustain some degree of perineal trauma during birth,[1] and the majority of these will need sutures to aid healing. The challenges when considering the needs of your hEDS client are around ensuring adequate anaesthesia, protection of the hips, choice of suturing material and methods, and prevention of further bruising or damage during the suturing process. The hEDS skin tends to be thinner, more fragile and more likely to bleed, so not only is it more prone to tearing during birth but the stitching process can be more bruising and the sutures themselves can tear through the skin more easily. In addition, the hEDS skin can take longer to heal and so aftercare and monitoring are even more important than usual.

The sooner the perineum can be checked for suturing, the better, and certainly within an hour – before the tissues start to swell, and to minimise any blood loss or increased risk of infection,[2] not to mention that this woman may really be wanting a shower and a tray of hot NHS tea and toast which, after giving birth, turns out to be, quite simply, the very best tea and toast of any new mum's life.

There appears to be a general consensus amongst hospital trusts that suturing should be delayed for an hour following a water labour or birth,[3] because the 'tissues need time to revitalise following prolonged immersion in water'[4] and, although there does not appear to be any evidence to support the notion that the tissues of the vulva and perineum in particular are affected by being in water for a long time (the area is naturally permanently moist, after all), there is some evidence that it can reduce the integrity of other body tissues[5] so, if your hEDSer has enjoyed time in the birthing pool and is not actively bleeding or concerning you in any other way, it seems prudent to hold off suturing even if you have examined the perineum quickly postnatally.

I have frequently seen mums asked to 'hand baby to your partner' during suturing. I cannot understand this at all. This newly introduced couple are up to their necks in endorphin soup and, if you leave them together, chances are that you will not need to give quite so much pain relief. Furthermore, feeding will often get going much more gently and easily if you are otherwise engaged and mum and baby can simply cuddle and muddle rather than being urged to 'latch and attach'.

So, once you have gathered all your suturing kit together, spent time explaining what needs to be done and gaining informed consent, get as much light as you can and help your client to be comfortable with their little one. You shouldn't need stirrups – they're not used in the home birth situation and they can be devastating for the hEDS hips. They also minimise the ability to fidget into a better, more limb-friendly position when half an hour in the same place is starting to take its toll. If stirrups are deemed essential for careful suturing then get as much help as needed to ensure the hips do not come under any undue strain.

How much local anaesthetic is needed will vary from hEDSer to hEDSer, and from day to day for that same mum, but anticipate needing the maximum amount and, potentially, Entonox®, focused breathing and the distraction of a feeding baby in addition. Some hEDSers get good anaesthesia from a normal amount of local, but it wears off very much sooner than you would expect, so keep plenty of lignocaine to hand for topping up.

*I discovered that, for me, hEDS and local anaesthesia don't mix: episiotomy and stitching up with no pain relief at all and I felt every stitch!*

Erif

*The epidural didn't work on me so they had to spend a lot of time numbing me with a local before they could start stitching. I warned them I had EDS and would need a lot, but the obstetrician was still stunned at how much I needed and how fast it started wearing off.*

Rhi

This is a woman who really needs non-absorbable sutures which can be left in for a fortnight if necessary, in order to fully heal. Absorbable sutures are more likely to break down and pull out of this fragile and slow-to-repair skin. Despite the NICE and Royal College of Obstetricians and Gynaecologists (RCOG) recommendations to use a continuous suture using absorbable material for perineal repair,[6] when it comes to your hEDS client, use interrupted stitches and a very low-tensile and soft material which is least likely to cause irritation or sensitivity. As discussed in Chapter 11, I favour black silk, which is incredibly soft, unlikely to irritate or cause an allergic reaction and is more likely to give if put under tension than pull through the skin.[7] This should have been thought about and planned for in advance – black silk or other non-absorbable sutures are rarely to hand in the maternity world but they can often be tracked down, given time and determination, from other departments such as orthodontic surgery.

*The hospital agreed to use black silk stitches for me as per my request since booking appointment. Planned a home birth, all was OK until the day the midwives tried to collect them from delivery ward. They point blank refused. The very best I was allowed was 'super strength purple stitches'. I declined the use of them with a grade 2 tear. I healed better than I expected.*

Zoe

A few stitches, placed gently and deeply, used to just hold the edges of the tear together with minimal tension and left in place long enough for healing to complete should be the aim.[8] It is almost impossible to explain the difference in experience between thin, rather wiry Vicryl™ sutures breaking down in the perineum and the thicker, yielding nature of black silk. The latter don't prickle or pull and the knots don't poke or catch on your sanitary towel. Sure, they have to be removed, but they can be removed individually, over days if necessary, as each part of the perineum closes securely, and I have yet to speak to an hEDSer who wouldn't rather have sutures that need to be removed than have their perineum break down as their sutures either dissolve or pull through their delicate skin.

Using a different material and method from usual should not be a big ask when compared to the trauma caused by the pain and distress of an unhealed perineum, but sadly, I have had far too many women tell me that their antenatal birth plan requests for securing non-absorbable sutures and being stitched carefully as described were ignored. No wonder hEDSers are an anxious bunch!

*The specialist unit I was under said that I needed silk stitches after birth. The hospital I gave birth at ignored that advice and stitched me with dissolvable instead. I ended up with wounds not healing, stitches not holding, eventually got an infection and had to be restitched.*

Steph

In view of the apparently increased risk of pelvic organ prolapse following episiotomy in this population[9] (although it is true that not all studies support this finding), if your hEDS woman has had an episiotomy, if there is an extended tear with the possibility of anal involvement, or if you are not completely confident about suturing using interrupted non-absorbable sutures, hand over to the obstetric team, ensuring that you explain the need for a particular approach with this client and thrust those silk stitches into their hands as you do it.

After checking that the repair is complete and that bleeding has stopped, a careful digital check of the anus along with adequate pain relief, and a thorough discussion, explanation and trial run of Kegel exercises should follow.[10] Remember that this community often face lifelong issues with bladder and bowel function, even in the absence of any births, so thorough perineal care and health are essential along with solid follow-up through the postnatal period.[11]

## Bladder Care

Women throughout the land seem to think that stress incontinence is simply part and parcel of having been pregnant and giving birth.[12] Knowing nods and winks, along with in-jokes about no longer being able to join the trampolining club or go for a jog oil the conversation at postnatal coffee mornings, and now even TV adverts seek to normalise 'leaking a bit of wee' by promoting pantie pads over eradicating the need for them!

Our patriarchal society doesn't help – a research bias towards men means that problems that more commonly impact women can fly under the radar or get dismissed.[13] Around a third of women suffer from stress incontinence after having a baby and this figure doesn't take into consideration other post-birth bladder dysfunctions such as incomplete emptying and recurrent UTIs. This represents a significant bladder morbidity in our postnatal population which could be greatly reduced with simple and early interventions.

The additional challenge when caring for a postnatal woman with hEDS is that her everyday experience of pre-pregnancy bladder behaviour may be quite off-kilter and so she may need extra guidance as to how to monitor and protect her postnatal bladder recovery. First, it is imperative that you know what normal is for her. She may be completely oblivious to the fact that either her frequency or her ability to go all day without feeling the need to pee are either unusual or potentially problematic in the postnatal period. Not feeling the need to empty a grossly over-full bladder might be great when you are hiking across the Yorkshire moors but could lead to a PPH in the hours following giving birth, and frequent trips to the loo may mask an inability to fully empty the bladder if the woman is unaware of that possibility. Of course, midwives and carers supporting that hEDSer need to know that just because she has no sense of an over-full bladder doesn't necessarily mean that she isn't in retention or have a very full bladder. Just because this new mum can reassure you that she always needs to pee five times an hour doesn't mean that there isn't now a new problem. Everyone needs to be on the ball in the immediate and longer postnatal period.

There is a natural diuresis in the hours immediately following birth which continues for a couple of weeks.[14] Ensuring that your hEDSer is carefully supported to use the toilet as soon after suturing as possible is essential, taking care to help her up very slowly and escort her all the way in case of a POTS episode leading to a fall. The first pee should be measured[15] and, if you have any concerns at all, continue to measure urinary output as well as blood loss, uterine contractibility[16] and bladder distension[17] for the next six hours and, as with any other woman, if minimal or no urine is passed in that time then catheterisation should be considered.[18] If there is a labour history of instrumental birth or epidural use, the catheter should be left in for at least 12 hours.

Following that first post-birth trip to the loo the frequently peeing hEDSer subgroup may benefit from guidance on how to improve the likeliness of fully emptying their bladder by doing some simple Kegel squeezes after they think they have finished and then trying again. Staying on top of their pain medication and sitting in a warm bath can also help, along, of course, with having privacy to prevent 'stage fright' inability to pee. If you feel confident enough in your own bladder palpation skills then consider teaching this skill to your hEDSer so that she can self-monitor.

The super-sized bladder subgroup should be advised to head to the toilet to pee every couple of hours whether they feel the need to go or not as a distended bladder may not cause this woman any pain at all but could predispose her to bleeding. As with her frequently peeing hEDS sister, ensuring adequate pain relief, warmth, privacy and bladder palpation skills can help this woman to take back some responsibility and autonomy in her own care.

## POTS

The hEDS population are a dizzy community[19] and it takes very little to trigger an episode – hunger, getting up too swiftly or simply not doing any exercise for a week. Giving birth can out-gun any of those relatively minor provocations and the dysregulation of the ANS can make recovery slower. The blood pressure may read normally but you might still see pallor and shaking in your hEDSer following birth. Lying down may help for a while but then, when she goes to get up again...

Meeting the need of the POTSy hEDSer is the ideal work of a birth partner or doula. Salts and fluids are the mainstay of managing POTS on a day-to-day basis along with regular exercise.[20] Ideally the tea and toast bonanza should have been sorted out during the suturing or, if suturing is not taking place immediately and there is no reason to wait, as soon as the examination of the third stage is completed. Isotonic drinks will help to keep a POTS attack at bay whilst waiting for the toasting bread to set off the smoke alarms (why are all NHS toasters set to 'cremate'?) and simple passive leg exercises can also help stave off dizziness for a short while.

As we have seen, POTS is not just about a racing heart and feeling dizzy – the entire ANS is prone to going AWOL as the body tries and fails to reach homeostasis when triggered. Along with the normal adrenaline shakes so commonly seen in the post-birth woman, the hEDSer may feel genuinely terribly cold, or chokingly hot, and sudden noises or movement may cause panic (see Chapter 8). Keeping her baby skin-to-skin in her arms will help mitigate against some of this, particularly the anxiety as the endorphins race through her body and start to ease her breathing.

A number of warmed blankets thrown over the skin-to-skin pair will help ease cold, whereas an unwarmed blanket will simply trap the 'always cold' hEDSer in her very own cold-bunker. In the home environment it is generally pretty easy to find a hot water bottle to warm towels and blankets ahead of time. In the hospital it can be a bit trickier, but a willing birth partner can shove a blanket or towel up their jumper during the second stage and pre-warm it.

The 'always hot' hEDSer may well need a fan on her whilst her baby has a warmed towel or blanket placed over their back and the back of their head, and the 'too hot, too cold' hEDSer needs both a pile of warmed blankets and a sturdy fan. This may seem like unnecessary luxuries but POTS symptoms can escalate if not managed, making the early postnatal hours a misery.

## Headache

Those with hEDS are very prone indeed to headache, with many in the community having it as an ongoing daily symptom.[21] There are a wide range of causes, from migraine to cranio-cervical instability and from food and medication sensitivities through to Chiari malformation (see Chapter 6). The hormonal fluctuations, changing hydration needs due to lactation, disturbed sleep and increased stress will potentially make the postnatal headache journey even worse, and we will explore this in the next chapter. In the immediate postnatal hours, however, midwives and other carers should be alerted to the increased risk of spontaneous cerebrospinal fluid leak in those with connective tissue disorders[22] and also in those who have recently used the Valsalva technique[23] so any positional or orthostatic headache, even in the absence of an epidural or spinal anaesthesia, should be flagged up for investigation swiftly.

> *I'd had a C-section. They said I had a post-lumbar puncture so fluid leaked from my spine to my brain and I suffered the worst headache for three days post birth. The only way I was OK was laying completely flat.*
>
> Faye

## Anaemia

It is thought that, in developed countries, somewhere between 20 per cent and 50 per cent of all postpartum women have an Hb less than 110g/l a week after birth and below 120g/l for the whole of the first post-birth year.[24] It is certainly arguable that the human female is perfectly evolved to regulate the Hb, adjusting it to changing needs throughout pregnancy and then replenishing iron stores after the birth but, as we saw in Chapter 9, the hEDS population have all the potential to be ticking along, unbeknownst to anyone, on chronically low iron stores even before they embark on pregnancy due to their increased likelihood of heavy periods,[25] easy bruising and frequent inflammation as a result of their regular injuries. Even in the absence of a PPH, there will be some blood lost during birth and postnatally and, when there are already chronically low iron stores, a relatively low to moderate loss can be the straw that breaks the camel's back.

Haemoglobin measurements can remain within normal levels even with low ferritin[26] – only dropping as the iron stores reach critical low – leading to fatigue, depression and the inevitable toll this can take on the building of a good mother–baby relationship. I wonder how many mothers are diagnosed with postnatal depression when they are, in fact, walking around with undiagnosed low iron stores.

Hopefully you have checked the serum ferritin levels at antenatal booking, treated where appropriate and have an idea of your hEDSer's pre-birth level, but, in any case, it is worth checking again soon after birth and flagging up if the results show serum ferritin levels less than 30µg/l so that appropriate treatment with either oral iron or parenteral iron can be started quickly.[27]

## Pain

The hEDS population live with pain – it is what initially marks out the hEDSer from those who are simply very supple in their joints – and the pains are often widespread and chronic. Pregnancy can lead to worsening of the pain symptoms as the joints become even more loose,[28] and then along comes the birth to pour even more fuel on the fire. Anyone who has laboured and given birth will recognise that feeling, in the first few hours and days, of aching in places you didn't know existed. The woman with hEDS will have all of those pains and then, potentially, some extra ones just for good measure.

In labour and birth the lax joints will have been able to move beyond the normal range without their owner being very aware of it – one of the reasons why it is so important for midwives and birth supporters to pay close attention to limb position during labour. Every time a limb or joint is moved out of range, little micro-injuries take place and it is the accumulation of all these micro-injuries that can lead to hEDS 'flares' (see Chapter 6). Little wonder that almost 40 per cent of hEDSers find that pain symptoms are worse postnatally.[29]

Longer-term pain management will be addressed in the next chapter but, even in the immediate aftermath of birth, it is important to bear in mind that the pain that your hEDSer is experiencing may be above and beyond the expected range for a postnatal woman and should be explored and taken seriously. The joints associated with labour and birthing – the hips, pelvis and coccyx – are likely to have taken the brunt of the forces and potentially been put through their paces a little too fast. Your hEDS mum will be more than capable of telling you if her hips have popped out at any point during birth but she may not know if the intense pain in her lower back and bottom is due to a strained, dislocated or fractured coccyx, or if her PGP symptoms which she became so familiar with in pregnancy are worse because her symphysis pubis has now stretched even more.

If she is staying overnight in hospital, this woman needs plenty of pillows to support her limbs in a natural position and a reminder to keep her legs hip width apart and parallel whenever she is sitting or lying – she simply won't always know where her limbs are because her proprioception is, frankly, pants! She may feel entirely comfy in a position which looks crazy but the damage being done may cause lasting pain. Mobilisation is so essential to this population to avoid deconditioning and a subsequent increase in symptoms that it is worth giving regular pain medication even if the hEDSer isn't particularly uncomfortable, whenever the drugs trolley makes an appearance, to ensure she can get up and about as often and as easily as possible.

A referral to the maternity physiotherapist team should be made as soon after birth as is humanly possible so that the hips, symphysis pubis and coccyx (as well as any other joints which might have taken a hammering during labour and birth) can be checked and a rehabilitation programme drawn up.[30] Being proactive rather than reactive will save time and precious NHS resources in the long run.

## Breastfeeding

The rates of breastfeeding in the UK are truly shocking – we have one of the very worst rates in the whole world.[31] I spent my entire midwifery life as a specialist in the field of infant feeding and, whenever I bemoan our atrocious record with colleagues they say that what women need is more support from their midwives and care assistants. But this simply doesn't stand up to scrutiny – every woman in the UK, unlike most other countries, has regular free access to a midwife in pregnancy and the early postnatal days, and I can put my hand on my heart and say that, of the many thousands of women I have supported when they have run into difficulties, not once have they said, 'If only one more midwife had shown me what to do!' Quite the opposite – they have felt utterly overwhelmed by the number of health care professionals who have come along and shown them. They complain about conflicting advice and quickly come to believe that it is themselves who have got it all wrong – midwives show them and show them and show them but, once the professional has headed off-duty, the baby and mum cannot seem to get things sorted. The sense of sadness, guilt and failure can hang around long after the baby has grown up and gone to school.

Women came out of their primitive shelters, blinking into the light, clutching their baby to their breast, gloriously oblivious to the words 'tummy to mummy, nose to nipple and wait for the big mouth!' They muddled their baby in for a cuddle in the pitch black of the first post-birth night, and the highly evolved baby with all its survival reflexes securely in place simply fussed and mushed about until they got on and got on with it. I have worked alongside women from right across the globe (mums and midwives) and they invariably pull me to one side and whisper, 'What is it with the UK and all those pillows and weird feeding positions?' Beats me, although I have witnessed with growing alarm the spread of the miserable and non-evidenced 'latching and attaching' fashion which bears no resemblance to the way women have snuggled their babies in to the breast since time began and continue to do in countries that have high rates of breastfeeding.

But let me climb down from my soapbox (when I have completed this tome and replenished my energy I shall write my book *Breastfeeding: How to Bung Your Baby on Your Boob with Your Eyes Closed!*) and simply tell you that, if you show your hEDSer the now-standard 'latching and attaching' you could be doing untold long-term harm to her joints. I have helped an hEDSer rehabilitate from a trapped nerve and a Bell's palsy caused by holding her baby in the cross-hold position for just one feed. Women without hEDS complain bitterly to me that the standard UK feeding holds are unsustainable and cause neck, shoulder and wrist pains as well as rolling the baby into positions that cause sore nipples as their little one tries, in vain, to remain securely anchored on the breast. The hEDSer, or any other mum for that matter, should never be expected to hold her arms up, pillow or no pillow, in what I call the

'Strictly Come Breastfeeding' hold – it actively inhibits normal baby-at-the-boob behaviour[32] and makes feeding a baby whilst eating a Curly Wurly much too tricky!

Immediately after birth, and for the first few days, mum should be supported with lying down to feed with a soft pillow under her head, baby pulled in really close, skin to skin and very low below the breast. Without needing to look but by feeling her baby's mouth deeply pressed against the underside of the breast, the wide mouth reflex will trigger and baby will reach back and up and faff their way on...as long as mum doesn't try to pull away to see what is happening but actively draws baby in closer as she feels the reflex kicking in. Yup – that big open mouth reflex is triggered by a deep touch and pulling away slightly to watch and 'wait for the big mouth' switches down the reflex and the mouth actually starts to close – now you know why so many mums today are told that their babies have 'such a little mouth!' Holding any position for more than a minute or two can be intensely uncomfortable for the loose-limbed hEDSer so she needs to be able to just relax, pretty much hands-free, and recover whilst her newborn enjoys the self-service café.

There has been a lot of confusion and anxiety over the past decade or so over the subject of co-sleeping, mostly due to the inclusion of incidences of sudden infant death syndrome (SIDS) in the presence of harmful sleeping behaviours.[33] There is such ample evidence that safe co-sleeping practices protect and prolong the breastfeeding journey that UNICEF, the Baby Sleep Information Source (Basis) and the Lullaby trust[34] all support informing mothers about how to co-sleep whilst reducing risks (see Figure 16.1).

In the immediate hours after birth, mothers are often wired but tired – lying awake gazing at their newest tribe member – and being separated, unable to easily reach their baby, is often described as being like having your right arm cut off. A clip-on bassinet, next-to-me crib or simply a cot brought right up to the edge of the bed can enable the new mother to stay close enough to touch her newborn when having them in their bed isn't possible or safe (for instance, when the woman is under the influence of narcotic drugs or her baby is premature). But, whenever and however possible, if your hEDS client can be supported to have her baby tucked in safely, she will be able to continue to support and rest her limbs and joints whilst soothing her peach-fresh bundle. I shall be eternally grateful to the gentle midwife who sat right through her night shift next to my bed – I woke up in the early hours to find her writing quietly and she said simply, 'I could see you had your little one in feeding and didn't want to disturb you so thought I would sit and do my work here and watch over you both!' That was a true gift!

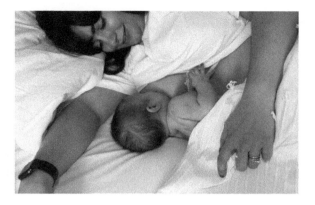

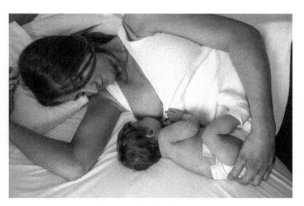

*Figure 16.1 Co-sleeping*

Women have always slept with their babies and will continue to do so whether or not they intend to, those breastfeeding hormones ensuring that they fall asleep as soon as the suckling begins, and mothers and professionals alike can be pointed in the direction of solid evidence-based information and guidance[35] so that they can make informed and safe choices which better reflect their own preferred style of parenting.

Many hEDSers are on a catalogue of medications and fret about being able to combine good EDS pharmaceuticals with breastfeeding.

They may make a needless decision to formula feed in order to be able to continue with their medication because there is a wealth of misinformation about drugs and mums' milk. The good news is that, for those who take the time to look, there are also little oases of calm and knowledge where you can get reliable advice from specialist pharmacists, so there is never any reason why a woman shouldn't be able to continue to feed her baby in the way she chooses.[36]

## Baby

EDS is an inherited condition in an autosomal, dominant manner.[37] So the baby of the hEDSer mum has, in theory at least, a 50 per cent chance of inheriting the condition. However, in practice, more girls than boys are diagnosed – probably because they are more likely, thanks to hormones, to be hypermobile and more symptomatic, so they flag up. This tends to allow affected boys to fly under the radar. Because their joints are more stable, they are less likely to have widespread joint injury and pain, and their other hEDS-related issues such as bladder and bowel problems along with allergies and anxiety (to mention just a few things in the hEDS bucket of fun) simply get treated independently and outside of the EDS framework.

All babies are more flexible than all adults so that they can fold up, origami-style, into the confines of a human womb, and all babies, as midwives all know, have dysregulated autonomic nervous systems and so, like the adult hEDSer, have poor thermoregulation, enthusiastic reflexes, whacky breathing and over-sensitive guts. So it can be virtually impossible to diagnose hEDS in the newborn infant. This does not mean to say that there is nothing that marks the hEDS baby out as different and about which it helps to be aware.

### Floppy Infant Syndrome

As midwives support a newly birthed mother to greet her newborn baby, they are already expertly assessing that baby's condition and behaviour. We talk about how a baby 'handles', simply knowing, through experience, how a baby feels in our hands when all is, or isn't, well. Tone is one of those markers, which is hard to define but easy to sense when you have handled enough babies and, when there is a lack of it, it is quite noticeable. The baby affected by hEDS, whilst not as likely to be as floppy as babies with rarer forms of the syndrome such as the kyphoscoliotic subtype, may still feel looser-jointed than an unaffected baby.[38] Just like their overly limber mums, they may have good muscle tone whilst lacking the strong collagen to help keep their joints more stable. As you pick up and handle this little one you may just sense the arms moving noticeably out of the normal range for a baby, or those legs may fly up for a nappy change just a bit too easily. As I say, a tricky one to explain but obvious to feel for the experienced baby-handing hands. Remember that every time joints move past the normal range, there is the potential for macro- and micro-damage, leading to pain later in childhood with all the implications for development and education that holds,[39] so take extra care, when examining this baby, to support those floppy limbs.

### Clicky Hips and Joints

Often these tiddlers are simply rather 'clicky'. The hips should be very carefully checked as clicky hips were found in 12 per cent of one hEDS study population (the rate in the general newborn population is around 2%–3%) and actual dislocation of the hips found in 4.8 per cent (the normal rate being 1%).[40] As this is an infant population notoriously late to crawl and walk even in the absence of hip dysplasia, early diagnosis and treatment is essential.

You might feel shoulder blades and ribs click a little alarmingly when you pick the baby out of the crib and the ankles are often a little clicky when lifted for nappy changes. It will be many years before a more formalised diagnosis of hEDS will be made, but it is important to note these little anomalies, and the possible reason for them, in the baby notes so that the baby can be properly assessed to exclude other diagnoses and so that the next person to hold the baby knows what to expect from this little bundle of 'Rice Krispies'.

### Skin

Newborn baby skin is fabulous – the smell and the soft, downy feel is just glorious. The skin of a baby with hEDS is on another level and can alert you to the truth that this baby has something more going on than simply a greater degree of limb laxity than most babies.[41] The skin itself is silky smooth and the lack of strong collagen underneath makes the flesh unusually yielding, so your fingers can sink in as they would into bread dough. The hair on the body as well as the head, also lacking robust collagen, can be extremely fine and soft – a trait that can continue right through the hEDSer's life. This skin can seem very fine and, because it can be so thin, the blood vessels in the skin beneath the eyes are more obvious, giving the appearance of dark circles.

## Bruising

These little ones can bruise![42] They may not be running around the house yet, ping-ponging through doorways like their mum, but they are still very prone to popping up a nice purple bruise from seemingly innocuous handling. Changing a nappy or holding the face whilst you check the eyes may be enough to cause a mark no matter how gentle you feel you have been, and, of course, if there has been a difficult or instrumental birth there may be more bruising than you would normally expect, so make notes of any bruises you notice as you check in these first few hours and days and counsel the parents very carefully on the importance of giving prophylactic vitamin K to their little one. I have only ever had to deal with one case of unusual bleeding in a baby in my midwifery career; the mother was very hypermobile and at her mother's request, baby had not had vitamin K. I arrived to do a home visit a few days after the pair had been discharged home and noticed a significant pseudo-menstruation which mum told me had been going on for a couple of days, and a few new bruises along with some fading ones. After an injection of vitamin K the bruising and pseudo-menstruation resolved quickly and there was no further bleeding. Of course, the hEDSer baby has, in all likelihood, the same level of clotting factors as their non-hEDS peers but the additional support from vitamin K in these early hours and days seems prudent.

## Cardiac Anomalies

The likelihood of an increased risk of cardiac anomalies in the client with hEDS is still debated and significant issues are rare in this group,[43] but there does appear to be a possible link with mitral valve prolapse in adult hEDSers[44] and so it is possible that, when you or a paediatrician comes to do the first paediatric examination, you notice a mitral valve murmur. Although it is unlikely to be of any great ongoing consequence, it should of course, if found, be followed up appropriately and swiftly. The genetics of collagen disorders is very complex with lots of over-lapping between various syndromes and, because cardiac anomalies such as valve insufficiency and dilatation of the aortic root can occur wherever collagen is weak, being proactive rather than reactive saves time, money and distress in the long term.[45]

## CHAPTER 17

# Going Forward

## Introduction

It is truly heartbreaking to hear how many women in the hEDS community say that they cannot face having another much-wanted baby because of the trauma they suffered first time around and the increased level of pain and other symptoms they suffered as a result. With really good, woman-centred care throughout pregnancy, labour and birth the chances of this woman coming out the other side feeling permanently broken should be greatly reduced. The story is not yet over, your job is not done – the ongoing journey into motherhood also offers opportunities for protection against future problems and, for the hEDSer whose body is already struggling as a result of her pregnancy and intrapartum experience, to repair some of the damage. For the majority of postnatal care, midwives and other health care professionals need not do or suggest anything different from that which they'd do or suggest with the general postnatal population. Here we will focus our attention on those areas that need a bit more of an hEDS perspective.

## Mum
### Schedule of Postnatal Care

Chat to your nan and your mum about their experience of postnatal care and the fast decline of provision becomes apparent. Over the course of just a couple of generations the average hospital stay following birth has fallen from almost a week to just a day or two at the most.[1] At the same time the number of home visits has also plummeted. Your nan would have expected to see a midwife every day for 10–14 days (twice a day for the first three days) whilst the 21st-century woman may well get just one or two home visits overall.[2] This is playing out at a time when, over the past 30 years, the number of caesarean section births has more than doubled.[3] So more than a quarter of women are recovering from major abdominal surgery at the same time as taking on care of a new baby and yet only getting a fraction of the professional face-to-face care their own mothers could have expected following birth.

Now, before we all start wringing our hands and bemoaning the death of good maternity care, it is notable that women remain, overall, consistently satisfied with their postnatal care. They appreciate being able to get home sooner to the comfort of their own bed and biscuit barrel. However, as happy as they are with the care they receive once home, they also wish that there was more of it, and there is evidence that moving to a more individualised approach may lead to less postnatal depression, improved rates of breastfeeding and greater maternal satisfaction overall.[4]

Although women prefer postnatal checks to take place in the home rather than in a hospital or clinic, in these days of tight budgets and staff shortages the global pandemic of COVID-19 at least taught us that, when we can't visit in person, a phone or video call is hugely appreciated and offers a good opportunity for supporting the newly birthed woman towards greater autonomy through self-monitoring.[5]

When it comes to supporting and protecting the hEDSer postnatally with her increased propensity for a wide range of physical and emotional challenges, consider an individualised plan combining a number of home visits to check the perineum and feeding, plus video or phone checks to ensure all other aspects of postnatal recovery are going as expected. This community is used to and proficient at monitoring the workings of their quirky body and so you can confidently expect them to relish the chance to check their own blood pressure and measure their own urine output if tasked to do so. Tell them what to look for and they will probably put their extra-long arms to good use, grab a mirror, and check their own stitches too.

*I asked for my notes and a post-birth debrief. I was told I should be grateful he was born healthy. Of course I am, but his birth left me with permanent pain and trauma – there's no reason I should be grateful for that. Mums should never feel like collateral damage after giving birth.*

Nina

## Stitches

Sutured carefully with non-absorbable, interrupted stitches, the hEDS perineum stands a good chance of fully healing.[6] Healing might take longer and the scar tissue itself may be atrophic.[7] Atrophic scars are set lower than the surrounding skin, are often wider than the original injury and thin in nature. They are very common in the hEDSer, with up to 46 per cent of those who had a caesarean section (CS) having abnormal CS scars.[8] The stitches should ideally be left in place for two weeks and, because these are interrupted sutures, they need not be all removed at once, so check carefully and be prepared to remove them over a series of days.

When we sit on our bottoms, the skin of the perineum stretches a little and this can create enough tension in the hEDSer's skin to cause the sutures to start to pull, so this is a lady who, having always been able to sit comfortably in the weirdest of positions, now needs to know how to sit...like a lady! Take a regular, soft bed pillow, folded in half down its length and place it at the very front of a chair or sofa. Get your client to sit back over it whilst holding it in place so that it ends up just under the lowest part of her thighs before they meet her knees. With her knees together, the pillow will tip her back just enough to take her off her sutured perineum but without transferring too much pressure onto her, possibly very bruised, coccyx. The relief is instantaneous and this is also an ideal position for feeding and changing a baby (see Figure 17.1).

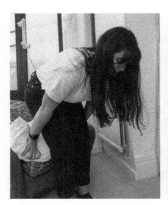 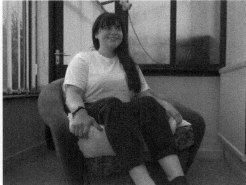

*Figure 17.1 Use of a pillow to relieve perineal pain*

Many decades ago it was thought important to keep stitches nice and dry to promote healing and so newly birthed mothers up and down the country were advised to have a daily bath and then warm and dry the perineum with a hairdryer. I'm delighted to say that the changeover to moist wound healing and the banning of hairdryers came after my four births and so I was able to enjoy that small daily pleasure. The good news for women is that studies now back up the original findings that dry heat on perineal wounds speeds up healing and reduces pain[9] and so the hairdryer – turned to the warm rather than the singe setting – can come back out to give poor, sore perineums another daily, blissful airing.

As with all postnatal women, using warm water to pour over the perineum after going to the loo and dabbing dry with a soft towel is better than using toilet paper and, when it comes to having the bowels open, supporting the perineum with a soft pad can reduce discomfort.[10]

The hEDS skin is genuinely very sensitive and easily irritated and chafed – no amount of pulping of sanitary towel material can stop it rubbing this woman's perineum and vulva, and even knickers can irritate. A better option for the hEDSer may be to go knickerless when at home and, whilst still bleeding, sit on soft towels or incontinence pads and then, when up and about, wear very soft washable period pants under loose clothing. The advice to wear loose clothes and 'go commando' may also be helpful for the long term as, interestingly, that is a popular self-help treatment for those who suffer from vulvodynia[11] and, of course, that tribe is rather over-represented in the hEDS community.[12]

## Pelvic Floor

Too weak, too strong...just like a high street coffee, getting the Goldilocks strength in the pelvic floor is never easy for the hEDSer. Years of trying to gain stability by constantly engaging the abdominal and pelvic floor muscles can lead to a hypertonic state in very many of us, which may go some way to explaining why there is more than six times the normal rate of vulval pain in this community.[13] At the other end of the scale, if the pelvic floor is not permanently 'switched on' the lax tissues can allow for an increased risk of incontinence and prolapse.[14]

Instructing your hEDS client to do plenty of pelvic floor squeezes might not actually be in her best interests if she already has hypertonic muscles. The hEDS population needs physiotherapy care throughout their life but physios who are deep in the hEDS geek are frustratingly hard to come by. Some of the bigger NHS hospitals specialising in rheumatology have specialist teams but outside of those areas physios are unlikely to specialise in the sheer array of issues suffered by this community.[15] However, physiotherapists working in the field of maternity will have a very good understanding of, and experience in, pelvic floor therapy and so ensuring that the hEDSer stays on the maternity physio books as she reaches term in her pregnancy rather than her being discharged and then having to go back on the waiting list seems sensible. Good pelvic floor health can have positive impacts on back and pelvic stability[16] as well as on coccydynia (pain in the coccyx), and, of course, on the normal functioning of the bladder and bowels. It is never too late to learn how to exercise the pelvic floor just the right amount in just the right way to achieve that Goldilocks strength.

## Bladder and Bowels

When we take care to protect the bladder and bowels by maintaining a clear bladder during labour, minimising perineal trauma at birth, and by closely monitoring and, when necessary, managing urinary output during those first postnatal hours, we reduce the risks of problems moment by moment and, importantly, we also pay forward, reducing the likelihood of ongoing maternal morbidity.[17]

As we have seen, the hEDSer is much more likely to enter pregnancy with abnormal bladder and bowel function.[18] Knowing what is normal for her is a good starting point postnatally, but then also teaching her what is normal for most other women and how she can monitor and improve her own function might go a long way to ensuring long-term health.

The hyper-stretchy-bladder contingent may well be unaware of their bulging bladder but acutely aware of the increasing backache and afterpains that a full bladder can cause. Teaching the woman how to palpate her bladder every hour or two and then, after peeing, to gently massage her fundus will kill a veritable handful of birds with one stone – preventing an overly full bladder, reducing afterpains[19] and also putting this new mum in touch with the workings of her bladder and womb.

The frequent loo-bothering section of the hEDS population may benefit from support to increase bladder capacity and improve pelvic floor function. It may be particularly tricky for this group to know where their 'normal' bladder issues end and their birth-induced problems start – that physio appointment cannot come soon enough for this woman.

For both tribes, completing a simple daily bladder assessment detailing whether the woman has urgency or lack of sensation, reduced flow or lack of flow control, or any pain at all when peeing can help her and you to monitor progress and alert you both to a problem.

*Both with my older child and my new baby, I've had to retrain my bladder – my bladder wasn't telling my brain it needed emptying. We're co-sleeping on the GP and HV's recommendation after I was getting less than two hours sleep in every 24 hours. However, co-sleeping is hard on my joints and I'm waking up with a lot of numbness and nerve pain in my arms. I'm hoping baby decides they like their next-to-me crib soon!*

Nicole

Bowel function after birth can take a few days to reassert itself but, come what may, at some point it really is a case of 'better out than in' and, given that the very thought of the first post-birth poo causes almost universal anxiety, it is astonishing that there is such a paucity of evidence detailing what does and doesn't help.[20] Bulk-forming medications which aim to soften the stool and to make it bigger may not help the women whose bowel simply refuses to shift stuff along, whilst a laxative might induce an episode of IBS. As we saw in Chapters 4 and 8, this is a tribe who are often dehydrated, who struggle to eat a varied diet, and might well be taking inadequate exercise. On top of this, they may be taking a variety of drugs including opiates even if they haven't had a caesarean section.

As with bladder function, it helps to know what is normal for this hEDSer whilst also bearing in mind that her 'normal' might actually be very abnormal and in need of improvement – just getting her back to how she was seems a low bar to clear. A good ongoing combination of regular fluid intake, a varied diet and getting a solid exercise routine in place is a good start. Her GP may need to review current pain medications before issuing a prescription for laxatives and consider recommending a range of non-pharmacological therapies such as CBT, mindfulness, acupuncture and massage instead. When reviewing pain scores it is important to bear in mind that the hEDSer may well have pain in her coccyx which could instigate or contribute to difficulty comfortably passing a stool,[21] so careful questioning is vital to get a full picture of what exactly is going on.

## Hydration

With their altered interoception and dysregulated ANS (see Chapter 8), the hEDSer can 'run dry' at the best of times and so, postnatally, needs to be extra-vigilant about maintaining hydration. She will most likely be used to taking on regular fluids and salt in an attempt to manage her POTS symptoms[22] but now needs to know that her fluid intake may well need to be even greater and, thirst not being her best guide, an increase in POTS symptoms despite having her usual intake may be more instructive.

## Diet

As with hydration, the hEDSer can have a somewhat erratic insight into her need for food[23] and is also more prone to feel grim if she skips a meal. She may well not realise she is hungry until it is too late, and then fill up too fast and before her true needs are properly met, only then to crash again before long. Three healthy meals and two nutritious snacks a day as a minimum will give that additional calorie cover for breastfeeding and stave off POTS attacks of nausea and shaking. It is often sensible to plan ahead and ensure that all the day's food is prepped the night before, and then eat by the clock rather than wait for those POTS symptoms to kick in as a brutal reminder to fuel up.

## Headache

Around 40 per cent of all postnatal women experience postnatal headaches.[24] A combination of head, neck and shoulder pain, this is one of the most common postnatal complaints and has a variety of causes from hormonal changes to stress, sleep disturbances and dehydration.[25]

The hEDS community suffer with chronic headache more than the general population and, of all the symptoms associated with hEDS, headache is right up there jostling for top spot.[26] Migraine alone is three times more common in this group and is experienced from an earlier age and in a more severe form.[27] Then there are many other forms of headache, mostly a direct result of the hypermobility in the neck and jaw. Head back to Chapter 6 for more detail on hEDS headache.

When assessing postnatal headache in your hEDS client keep in the back of your mind that this is a woman with an increased risk of cerebrospinal fluid leaks,[28] and that these can be triggered by spinal anaesthesia and also undue exertion such as using Valsalva during second stage.[29] Of course, the more likely causes of her headache are the same as for the non-hEDSer but it pays to be alert, at least, to the possibility that there may be more going on.

The headache resulting from a leak of cerebrospinal fluid normally occurs in the first 72 hours after dural puncture and is characterised by a frontal or occipital headache that is worse when sitting or standing, coughing or straining, and improves on lying down. In addition, there may be neck stiffness, nausea, vomiting, visual disturbances, light sensitivity and auditory symptoms, such as hearing loss, increased sensitivity to sound, and tinnitus.

Bed rest and extra fluids are no longer recommended for treating post-dural puncture headache (PDPH),[30] but adequate pain relief is essential until an effective blood patch, if required, is in place.

## Lochia

Most women I speak to seem to think that their lochia is loss from a bleeding placental site rather than endometrial shedding. The hEDSer who is 'a bit of a bleeder' can naturally worry that she will bleed more than the average bod, especially if she has a long history of heavy periods, so needs plenty of reassurance that if she keeps her bladder from overfilling and breastfeeds freely she is no more likely than any other woman to bleed more heavily or for longer. She may, of course, bleed from a slow-healing perineal tear or from haemorrhoids, but her lochia should be entirely normal and she should simply monitor her loss and flag up any concerns in the same way as her non-hEDS friends.

## Deep Vein Thrombosis

Deep vein thrombosis remains a leading cause of direct maternal death[31] and is five times more common postnatally than during pregnancy.[32] Caesarean section birth and PPH increase the risk of a woman developing a clot, and preterm premature rupture of membranes, although not itself a risk for developing one, does appear to increase the risk of death from a DVT.[33] Your hEDSer is, as we have seen, no more likely to need a caesarean birth than a non-hEDSer but, if she has had a C-section, she might well be finding it harder to mobilise due to increased pain sensitivity[34] and ongoing PGP and, in addition, she may well have lost more blood than average and had a pre-labour, pre-term SROM. Whether this woman has had a surgical or vaginal birth, whilst strongly plugging the message that, even more than any other new mum, she really does need to get back to daily activity and exercises (even if it is simply daily stretches),[35] you need to be alert to the likelihood that this woman's hips and pelvis might be extremely stiff and sore and so, until she is able to exercise as much as she should, passive leg exercises have to be slotted into the daily routine along with wearing some well-fitted TED stockings. If the hEDS mum has been prescribed heparin then she and you need to be prepared for the potential for heftier bruising and to monitor more closely for signs of abnormal bleeding.

## Anaemia

A lifelong bruiser and bleeder and with a history as long as your arm of digestive issues, this is a woman who desperately needs a full check-up of her iron stores before discharge from your care. Head back to Chapters 9 and 16 and you will see that haemoglobin levels can stay pretty normal whilst iron stores steadily drop, and then a relatively moderate bleed can tip a patient over the edge without warning.[36] Hopefully you were able to take blood antenatally for ferritin levels alongside the ubiquitous full blood count so will have some idea of the baseline before labour, but do it again before discharge and, even before results are back, make sure that your hEDS mother knows the basic dos and don'ts around diet and iron uptake, especially that she should avoid tea, coffee and calcium-rich foods such as dairy at least an hour either side of an iron-rich meal or taking any iron supplements.[37] These foods bind with iron, preventing full absorption, whilst vitamin C in fruit and juices enhances the uptake.

Ongoing iron deficiency (with or without a normal haemoglobin) can cause fatigue, exercise intolerance and depression as well as tinnitus and headache. Your hEDSer probably already ticked most, if not all, of these symptoms before pregnancy and now needs all the help she can get to avoid getting worse.

## Fatigue

All new mothers talk about sleep or, more precisely, the lack of it. In the years leading up to having their first baby, at every opportunity a woman's friends will tell her, 'Just you wait for the sleepless nights!' and it still comes as a surprise when they discover that their own baby, like every other baby on the planet, is highly evolved to require maximum attention during the hours of darkness.

It is a source of ongoing frustration for me that our society seems to fetishise a certain way of sleeping and pathologise anything sleep-wise that doesn't conform. Needless to say, the considered norm for sleep patterns is not one typically experienced by fertile women and certainly not the one that all new mothers are familiar with. From the menarche onwards, women sleep differently according to what is happening in their hormonal cycles[38] and they are encouraged to see these natural monthly differences as disordered and in need of managing and medicating back to a rather male model rather than, quite simply, the way hormonal women sleep. Likewise when a new baby joins the household, women are constantly made to feel that their new normal is not normal at all when, of course, women and babies have evolved together over the millennia to survive broken nights perfectly well – their sleep should be viewed as different and requiring a slight lifestyle change rather than being aberrant and problematic.

Those with hEDS typically experience sleep very differently. Aside from sleep being affected by pain, alterations to the functioning of the autonomic nervous system can impact on how hEDSers fall asleep and stay asleep, as we saw in Chapter 8, and, as a result, they complain a heck of a lot about being tired.[39] Happily, this also means that many of the community have learnt various strategies for coping and so come to motherhood either as proficient nappers or accepting of their permanently 'tired but wired' existence.

What the hEDS postnatal mother needs to know is that the so-called lack of sleep faced by all new mothers is actually just a completely different but not abnormal way that women have evolved to sleep so that they can protect and care for their baby overnight whilst still achieving enough deep, restorative sleep. By ensuring that they continue (or begin) to schedule in a daily nap and have a couple of 'quiet times' in the day, they really will be OK and, very possibly, their deep sleep being protected by breastfeeding hormones, be better than they were before getting pregnant.

An open and supportive conversation about safe co-sleeping can be a genuine game changer for any new mum and even more so for the hEDSer whose joints will struggle to get them in and out of bed to lift, soothe and endlessly rock a baby who is pre-set to need constant in-arms security.[40] To deny the reality of the lived experience of night-time mothering and insist that women abstain from behaviours that protect the feeding and caring relationship simply forces women to lie to health care professionals about their co-sleeping habits which, in turn, cuts them off from conversations about how to do it safely and comfortably.

Reframing our own professional conversations around postnatal, new-mum sleep by normalising rather than pathologising the different experience we all have of those nighttime hours for at least a couple of years after giving birth can empower women to stop seeing themselves as broken and to start exploring practical strategies for living with a baby.[41]

## Pain

The joint and muscle pain that is a significant part of every hEDSer's life tends to get worse in pregnancy as a result of both hormonal changes and increase in weight.[42] The neck, back, pelvic girdle, knees, ankles and wrists can all take a bit of a hammering over the nine months and it is very unlikely that the extra pregnancy pain will magically evaporate immediately after birth and now there are extra stressors for the body to deal with – lifting a baby, pushing a pram, and so on. We will explore ways to handle a baby in a more hEDS-friendly way further on in this chapter but, for now, let's remind ourselves that chronic prenatal pain can increase the risk for postnatal chronic pain and also for postnatal depression.[43] A review of pain medication, taking into consideration any contraindications with mum's milk, should be a priority to ensure this woman, whose body relies on staying conditioned, can get up and into a daily exercise routine before the ink is dry on the birth certificate. Extra rest is never going to help the super-bendy body so, no matter how loud the protesting, the hEDSer has to do whatever it takes to get back in the swim of things...literally!

Aside from pharmacological help, physiotherapy, daily stretches and exercise, other things that can help include warm baths, meditation, massage and orthotic supports. Well-fitted shoe insoles can relieve the pressure on the back, knees and hips as well as ankles and should be checked following birth because of the changes that feet can undergo during pregnancy.[44] A soft abdominal support such as Tubigrip® (worn over a light vest if skin sensitivity to the elastic is an issue) can help ease the abdominal aching associated with a diastasis recti, although only time and exercise will actually reduce the separation.[45] Futuro™ splints are great for limiting wrist movement whilst allowing normal finger grip and so can help those hEDSers with carpal tunnel syndrome[46] and can be combined with pain-relieving topical gels such as ibuprofen or diclofenac to reduce inflammation.

Many hEDSers have a stockpile of orthotic supports, splints and braces and each has their place for easing painful joints during an acute flare, but long term they risk deconditioning the body and increasing the likelihood of injury and pain – there is simply no substitute for regular exercise and for using whatever strategies make that exercise possible.

There are numerous complementary therapies on offer now which claim to reduce pain and increase mobility, from food supplements through to acupuncture and myofascial release, but most require time and financial investment, which can be in short supply to a new mum on maternity pay. However, many hEDSers will swear that one or other of them has proved helpful and, although the evidence on efficacy rarely glows and is often, at best, patchy, it isn't totally absent in all cases and so, you pays your money and you takes your choice.[47]

### Anxiety and Panic

Head back to Chapter 8 on the autonomic nervous system and you will see that anxiety and panic are pretty much endemic in the hEDS community, and have a rather different basis to the anxiety and panic diagnosed in the general public.[48] The hypervigilant ANS kicks in at the slightest provocation and then overcompensates when trying to reassert homeostasis, leading to a nausea-inducing switchback ride through life.

Approximately 20 per cent of women will suffer with anxiety postnatally, and somewhere between 3 and 12 per cent antenatally.[49] When we think of clinical depression it is easy to think of a picture of someone lacking energy and with a sense of hopelessness whereas for very many, and particularly in the context of childbirth, the symptoms are of overwhelming worry and fear, often in relation to the baby.

The experience of new motherhood for most women is a complex mix of joy and terror – 'Wow – look what I have done!' and 'Oh heck – what have I done?' There can be a minute-by-minute bubbling worry about interpreting, understanding and meeting this tiny creature's physical and emotional needs and, for the hEDSer, there is the additional worry about the short- and long-term impact having a baby will have on her body and mind, along with wondering what she might have passed on to her child in the way of a genetic legacy. It is natural for women to be worried and to be worried about their worry – to fear that their anxiety will have a negative impact on their child and on their relationship with their child – but, if strategies are put in place early in the postnatal period, then there is no reason at all to assume that a good attachment and bonding won't take place.[50]

Anxiety and panic in the hEDSer are tied up with their pain and poor proprioception as well as with their dysregulated ANS and faulty interoception,[51] so a multi-pronged approach is likely to be most helpful. Ensuring adequate pain relief (pharmacological and non-pharmacological), a solid return to daily exercise, and good care from a maternity physiotherapist as discussed above can be securely underpinned by counselling, CBT and mindfulness meditation, and I would argue that CBT and mindfulness, in particular, should be an automatic part of the hEDS treatment plan.

Once learnt, using CBT to reframe and challenge anxious thoughts and 'talk down' panic puts the power firmly back in the hands of the woman and reduces the need for antidepressants in this medication-sensitive population.[52] Furthermore, for the time- and money-poor new mum, CBT can be accessed online with or without additional counselling.[53]

Sitting alongside CBT as its newer cousin is mindfulness meditation[54] which, like the elder statesman, has the benefits of being available to the user day and night, free, and available online or, better still, on a smartphone app.[55] Both CBT and mindfulness can be hauled out in the twinkling of an eye to calm nerves, ease pain and manage an array of hEDS symptoms from tinnitus to POTS, and can become part of the daily routine during feeds, naps and walks. For the hEDSer, there needn't be any wait for a diagnosis of postnatal depression before helping her to access CBT and mindfulness, as clients can self-refer for NHS talking therapies and CBT[56] and can easily download one of the many excellent mindfulness apps and start benefitting immediately from some gentle meditation.

## Breastfeeding

There is absolutely no reason why the hEDS mum should not be able to breastfeed for as long as she wishes. Far from having hormonal problems, her body often responds rather strongly to hormones[57] – certainly my experience of working with this community is that the hEDSer often has an abundance of milk! Suckling a baby helps both mother and baby to relax and rest,[58] soothes the anxious mind and sore body with endorphins and oxytocin, may reduce the risk of PND[59] and can improve attachment and bonding.[60] Seriously, what's not to love about breastfeeding, especially in this sore, over-anxious, over-tired, hyper-lactating tribe?

The main challenge for breastfeeding when it comes to the hEDSer is around holding the baby and fatigue. Take a dive back into the previous chapter and you will find me hollering from my soapbox about the aberrant way we 'teach' women to hold their babies for feeding. Hopefully I convinced you to leave your breastfeeding hEDS client alone a little more in these first postnatal hours to rest alongside her new baby and do what women have always done – get to know each other gently and without pressure, allowing the baby to express its own natural and highly evolved rooting and latching reflexes without a 'back seat driver' getting in the way and causing a crash! Lying down to feed allows mum to rest and relax her bruised joints and perineum, and baby to stay warm and discover feeding at a more baby-shaped, unhurried pace.

There comes a time when mums simply have to feed sitting up or walking around or whilst opening the door to the delivery driver, and the hEDSer needs to be doing this in a way that uses her arms and hands as little as possible. It is notoriously difficult to describe with words how to bring a baby into the breast but take a look at Figure 17.2 and you will see that we can simply get comfy and then bring a baby in until they are pressed against us and let baby do the rest. Need a rhyme to replace 'tummy to mummy' and 'latch and attach'? Try 'cuddle and muddle!'

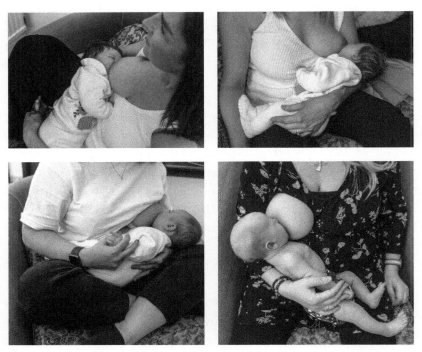

*Figure 17.2 hEDS-friendly 'cuddling and muddling' holds for breastfeeding*

Once snuggled in for time at the breast, the hEDSer needs reminding to fidget frequently and to check that her limbs and joints are in 'safe' positions by actively looking rather than relying on feeling – the pain from a twisted joint may well not hit until some time later and the damage could be significant.[61]

Feeding bras need to be extra-soft with no seams over the nipples, and it is worthwhile using soft cloth pads to quickly dry and warm the nipples after feeds to prevent an attack of Raynaud's syndrome, which affects almost 40 per cent of hEDSers.[62] Nifedipine can be given for intransigent cases of nipple vasospasm without any impact on the baby's well-being or mum's lactation,[63] but the simple home remedy of warmth and drying nipples works well enough for most women[64] and it is easy enough to buy heated gel pads to wear inside the bra whatever the season.

The tissue being so easily bruised 'like a peach' and slower to heal in the hEDSer, this new mum needs to care for her nipples during feeds even more than most mothers. Another great reason for encouraging her to cuddle her baby in a more 'historical' and evolutionarily authentic way is that the baby leading the way is more likely to adopt a position that allows for easier feeding, which tends to lead to comfier nipples – from an evolutionary perspective, positions that make feeding so unbearable as to render it impossible simply don't figure. There is a good chance that the nipples may be longer and stretchier due to the softness of underlying connective tissue, which can be helpful, but they can also sometimes get sort of caught up in the roof of the mouth on their journey to the far reaches of the baby's palate and get bad friction burn. This can be overcome by showing the mum how to actively and very quickly thread her nipple up and over the baby's tongue and to the back of its mouth for safe-keeping. It is easy when you know how and takes only a little practice. If nipples do get sore then drying them gently before squeezing out a small amount of breastmilk onto them is the simplest, and possibly the most effective treatment for the nipples[65] (unless there is a suspected thrush infection), as well as being more enticing for the baby when they next fancy cuddling in. As tempting as it is to recommend the latest cream or ointment on the market, it is best to steer away from creams and ointments with too many ingredients or with lanolin (no matter how purified it claims to be) due to the increased risk of sensitivity and allergy in this community.

Along with a potentially great supply, those with hEDS often seem to have a very enthusiastic let-down reflex – maybe due to the strong response to hormones, maybe due to dysfunction within the breast connective tissue impacting the contractions that occur within the breast[66] (I suspect the former) – and, due to altered interoception, this mum might find the experience far more intense and need reassurance that there really is nothing wrong.

*My milk came in hard, so I had to sleep with a size 1 nappy on each boob and on towels to not swim in milk at every feed.*

Nadia

Daily breast care using reverse pressure softening to reduce any engorgement will keep the breasts comfier without the danger of further increasing lactation, which massage towards the nipple, 'duct clearing' and expressing can cause.

With this tsunami of milk thrown at the baby with an almighty let-down reflex, you should not be surprised if the baby is a noisy feeder at times – gasping and spurting back milk as if being forced to drink a yard of ale at speed. The nappies may tend towards the greener spectrum of the rainbow – think passion fruit pulp rather than wholegrain English mustard and you will be on the right path. People do love to get in a real pickle about green poo but, if a baby is having plenty of wet nappies each day, is otherwise well and is growing as expected then there really isn't a problem and parents simply need reassurance. Sure, the baby may getting a greater proportion of foremilk than hindmilk than might otherwise be the case, but this doesn't mean they are getting too much foremilk and not enough hindmilk. I assure you that I can manage a stash of salad and still eat my own body weight in potatoes.

If the baby has inherited hEDS then it is worth noting that this is a baby tribe who can appear constipated even when exclusively breastfed, and this can catch out even the most experienced of us – it certainly had me scratching my head with my second son who, after the first month of life, would poo just once a fortnight and then it would be like very thick toothpaste! I had never come across this in the exclusively breastfed baby and it was only when I consulted with the EDS team in London that I was given the explanation that solid, rarely seen stools (once every 10–14 days) in the exclusively breastfed baby is a sign of EDS. Well, every day is indeed a school day! No treatment is needed in these cases, just reassurance for mum to keep suckling her baby freely and to be aware that, once on family foods, extra care may be needed to ensure 'true' constipation doesn't take hold. In the meantime…save money on nappies!

A medication review will have taken place antenatally to ensure any drugs were safe in pregnancy. As a good rule of thumb, any pharmaceuticals that are safe in pregnancy are even safer in breastfeeding – the breast being a less leaky 'sieve' than the placenta – but, if in any doubt, make sure to consult specialists in the field rather than relying on your or the GP's copy of the British National Formulary (BNF), which is not a robust guide for medications in mum's milk. Jack Newman,[67] The Breast Feeding Network (BFN) drug line,[68] Wendy Jones[69] and Tom Hale[70] all provide excellent and easy-to-access information for parents as well as health care professionals and help to protect the feeding relationship. Note that opiates such as codeine are no longer felt appropriate for use alongside breastfeeding because of the potential of a mum to be an unknown 'super-metaboliser'.[71] In any case, as I have already discussed a couple of times in previous chapters, opiates should not be a first-line choice of analgesic in hEDS due to their lessening effect on smooth muscle, the bowels and the respiratory centre in the brain.[72]

In conclusion, although many within the hEDS new mum community worry about their ability to breastfeed their baby, concerned that it might worsen their pain and sleep and pose a danger to their baby through medication transfer, they can be reassured and encouraged to see breastfeeding as a great addition to their hEDS list of helpful strategies.

*I had problems breastfeeding; his latch was good but it hurt and I was always so pinched. He had a posterior tongue tie and I was told it wouldn't be an issue but clearly it was. With the constant strain from everything baby-wise my hEDS flared. My pregnancy was OK pain wise but postpartum I broke. I had to put wrist splints on every time I wanted to pick up my son or feed him, but it got so bad when he was a month old that I wasn't able to pick him up or give him a bottle for a whole month. This still makes me cry to think about it.*

Anna

## Baby Care

Carrying, changing, bathing and generally caring for a baby all day and night is exhausting emotionally and physically. Relentless doesn't quite cover it at times. For women who struggle to hold a hairdryer for more than a few minutes without needing to take a break it can seem impossible. But babies have to be cared for: I remember an exhausted conversation with my own mum when she had come to rescue me six weeks into new motherhood and deep in the three-month colic phase of life, with a husband holding down an incredibly demanding job, working long hours to support his new family. As she marched up and down with my son over her shoulder, patting his backside so firmly that he had a little body-bounce each time, she declared, 'See, Rachel – he's quiet now. He is absolutely fine and you really don't need to worry!'

'But look at you, mum – you're marching up and down, patting and rocking him and not stopping at all and, every time you stop...he wakes and cries!'

'SO???' demanded my mum.

'I just cannot do that 24/7!' I protested.

A clang of silence and then... 'Well, what are you going to do then?'

As cruel as it seemed at the time, it woke me up to the reality that a baby is just perfect at being a baby and requires no mending. You really can't cure a baby of being a baby and so have to respond to their beautifully evolved needs in the best way that you can and stop running away from the reality, hoping that your baby will somehow turn into that unicorn 'by-the-book baby'.

The hEDSer needs practical solutions which meet her baby's need for constant close soothing whilst also protecting her own joints, mental health and need for rest. It simply has to be made possible and that is all there is to it. Support from family and friends is all well and good but, in the first three to four months of life, babies are highly evolved to settle best with their primary carer[73] – in this case, your hEDS client.

Slings are a fabulous creation and their use has been shown to go back to at least the last ice age.[74] Whilst the hEDSer is likely to have long arms and bendy, dexterous fingers, battling with a piece of material three metres long and requiring half an hour and a degree in origami to put on at the same time as trying to soothe a babe in arms is too much to ask. Nor should women be expected to take out a second mortgage to buy such a thing when they can be shown how to use a simple shawl or even a zipped-up jacket to keep their baby close and safe. Ticking off the T.I.C.K. checklist of safe sling use[75] should run alongside making certain that the shoulders and back are not being pulled out of alignment, remembering that proprioception is poor in this population and joints pull out more easily. The ideal is to have a wrap or sling that allows access to the breast for hands-free feeding whilst also negating or reducing the need to be pushing pushchairs and prams. There are plenty of sling libraries around the UK now so your hEDSer really should spend time test-running a variety of slings and wraps before selecting one that best suits her needs and her body.[76]

> *Feeding in a sling or carrier has saved me so many times when it's been way too painful to pick up or hold baby.*

Lauren

Protecting her own joints and back when lifting baby into and out of the sling also has to be considered, and it may help for mum to practise a few times in front of a mirror to compensate for her whacky proprioception. Bending down to a baby with the back held straight as the knees bend carefully, drawing baby in close to the body and then standing up and manoeuvring is safer than picking up a baby at arm's length. The car seat should be left in the car and baby lifted in and out (without twisting the body), rather than trying to pull out and carry a loaded seat – carrying even normally manageable weights on stretchy hEDS arms can strain every tendon and we can feel our joints lengthening and pulling apart.

Pushchairs and prams are fine as long as they are a good height, a doddle to put up, put down and lift, and are easy to push. This is a very high bar to clear, it seems, but there are products on the market that manage this feat, some of which are motorised for extra joint protection.

Bathtime can be kept to once or twice a week,[77] at least until the tot takes up mud wrestling, and, from a joint-preserving point of view, it can be easier and more soothing for all if mum simply takes baby in the bath with her whilst someone else is around to help. Babies can be fed at the same time as getting washed in the bath with mum, the deep, warm water easing joints and calming the overactive hEDS senses. When this is not possible, baby bathing can either be undertaken by the partner or another support person, or done in the kitchen sink with mum seated on a comfy stool, at the right height (see Figure 17.3). It just requires a little creative thinking.

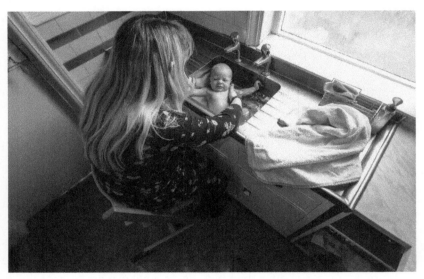

*Figure 17.3 Bathing baby seated at the sink*

Those with hEDS should learn to sit down and change a nappy on their lap (see Figure 17.4) which is, to my mind, the easiest way for all mums to do it anyway, and enables mums to feed one end at the same time as changing the other – remember those ads for shampoo which promised 'no more tears!'? Well, I give you my 'no more tears' version of nappy changing...you're welcome!

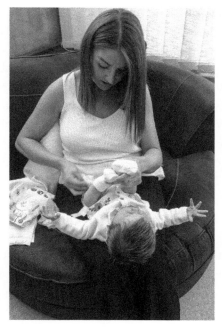

*Figure 17.4 Changing baby on the lap*

## Baby

Mums with hEDS fear their children inheriting their condition. Often seen as relatively benign to the outsider, hEDS can bring such a daily burden of symptoms that many women question whether to get pregnant at all. For those who do decide to tread the path of motherhood, their experience of feeling disbelieved or dismissed as neurotic is often repeated when their child shows signs of inheritance and, yet again, they struggle to get validation, diagnosis and support.[78] (A negative gendered bias has surely to be suspected when we consider that 72 per cent of affected men are diagnosed before the age of 18 as opposed to only 47 per cent of affected women, despite women generally being more musculoskeletally affected.[79])

In fairness, it can be tricky to diagnose hEDS in babies and young children because they are naturally more flexible than adults and the aches, pains and other symptoms tend to develop over years. But early diagnosis is important to ensure proper strategies are put in place before problems emerge or the child starts nursery. The hEDS mum is generally a savvy beast and knows only too well that as well as causing all the issues with joints, internal bodily system functioning and dysregulation of the ANS, hEDS has a strong associative relationship with attention deficit hyperactivity disorder (ADHD) and autistic spectrum disorder (ASD),[80] and this can weigh heavily on the already anxious mind.

In time she will need to face up to explaining to child minders and nursery care workers about her child's easy bruising and clumsiness, in the absence of a formal diagnosis. For now, though, the best this newly birthed hEDS mum can do is simply relax and know that, if her little one does turn out to one of the 50 per cent of 'lucky winners' in the great hEDS inheritance tombola she will be the perfect person to understand and support them.

So what are the things you might notice in these very early days and weeks which should be noted down as evidence for any future hEDS assessment?

### Tone

You may well have noticed the looser limbs of an hEDS baby at birth but, if you weren't around, then you may very well start to notice it now. This alert, perfectly normal baby can feel so unusually floppy.[81] Not the floppy of a poorly, worrying baby but a sort of toned floppiness. You pick them up naked and everything feels so yielding – that soft, super-squidgy flesh around joints which, although muscularly toned, move further than you are used to. The elbows, shoulders and knees seem a little disconnected and, as you handle this baby you will not be surprised to learn that tots with hEDS tend towards later crawling and walking[82] – the crawling stage is often bypassed altogether, and this topic forms a common dinner party conversation amongst hEDSers.

The hEDS mum should take care to carry her baby and put it into the crib with the limbs in 'normal' non-hyper-extended positions – just like her, even though the limbs *can* move well outside a safe range doesn't mean that they should be allowed to and, as tempting as it is to show off just how limber this baby is, every move outside the healthy norm can cause micro-traumas to store up. Highlighting her hand-held notes and notifying the health visitor that extra care needs to be taken when handling baby will protect this mum from the potential of yet more 'neurotic' labels being ascribed.

There are plenty of motor skill issues to face as the child grows up, from altered sitting postures through to difficulty with handwriting,[83] but rather than fret endlessly about the future, the anxious hEDS mum needs support to take one wobbly, ping-ponging step at a time.

## Bruising

There have been some high-profile cases of misdiagnosis of abuse in babies and children with EDS[84] and there is understandable anxiety around this in the EDS community.[85] For the hEDS baby the most likely issues are bruising and dislocation, with bruising being the more common unexplained symptom you will see. Something as simple as holding a baby's face between your fingers to check or clean their eyes might result in bruises, and you should take extra care when taking blood for the neonatal blood spot screening in the first week of life to minimise squeezing, and to accurately record the procedure in the notes.

Of course, with bruising can come jaundice, so babies that have had a difficult ride into the world or are premature should be monitored closely. The common practice of 'topping up' the jaundiced, breastfed baby simply doesn't have evidence to support it,[86] so unless phototherapy becomes necessary, continuing close, in-arms parenting alongside free access to the breast to ensure adequate hydration should be encouraged. Even when phototherapy is needed, supplementary fluids (oral or IV) offer no benefit and, in the sensitive hEDS baby, formula brings the risk of future allergy.

## Clicking

Your hEDSer will be used to her own clicking but it can still be alarming when it happens every time you pick your baby up. You may hear and/or feel little clicks in the baby's back, ribs, arms...anywhere really where bones align. Immediately after my fourth son was born, I lifted him up onto my chest to get a better look and felt a series of clicks in his body. My immediate thought (remember I have hEDS so my default button is set to 'panic') was that he had brittle bone disease and I was actually too shocked to say something. Very quickly my CBT kicked in and I reassured myself that the most likely explanation was that this was a 'bendy' just like his mum, but I have never forgotten the feeling of that little body crackling away in my hands, and of the spark of fear.

You need to know that these clicks are normal for the hEDSer and simply a result of the lax joints pulling apart and creating a tiny cavity (a process known as tribonucleation)[87] and sounds worse than it is. There is no evidence that, in the absence of dislocation, any long-term damage comes from joint cracking. If you find yourself handling a little 'Rice Krispie' baby, simply note down which joints appear to click and reassure mum.

Of course, these clicks are different from those heard and felt with 'clicky hips' and, if you notice any obvious signs of hip clicks or slides which haven't already been noted during the initial paediatric exami-nation, then you will need to make the necessary arrangements for this to be followed up as swiftly as possible. Carrying a baby in a well-fitted sling can help support the hips as they develop,[88] particularly those abiding in a bendy body, and as discussed above, makes life as an hEDS mum a little easier.

### Tongue-Tie

There appears to be a paradoxical finding in relation to the oral frenula in the hEDS baby. I have seen it stated that there is often an absence of the lingual frenulum[89] but, as a bit of a tongue-tie geek who is trained to assess and divide them and has published on the topic,[90] I suspect that in many cases where there is apparently no frenulum under the tongue, it is there but just very posterior.[91]

Now I am no fierce advocate for frenulotomy as it happens – the vast majority of babies sent my way with a suspected 'tongue-tie' simply had a very obvious frenulum (a perfectly normal part of the anatomy) and mum had been shown feeding techniques which would defeat the best of babies. Even with frenula that really do pull the tongue out of its natural flow of movement, most babies adapt to their favourite boob very happily if not pressurised to 'latch and attach'. But just occasionally there is a frenulum that is so fibrous, tight or impactful that frenul-otomy can protect an otherwise doomed breastfeeding relationship.[92]

If you suspect that there is a frenulum negatively impacting on your hEDS mother and baby's breastfeeding journey then, even if you cannot see a frenulum, get a good specialist to do a thorough examination and, if a frenulotomy is assessed to be appropriate seek a practitioner who will do a full division.[93] That sounds obvious, but many practitioners do a partial frenulotomy to 'just snip a little bit and see if that helps'. To me this is equivalent to doing a partial tonsillectomy and risk leaving behind the troublesome part, necessitating yet another procedure at a later date with all the associated risks.

### Autonomic Nervous System

Babies have dysregulated ANS. Midwives know that – it is why we are so keen for new parents to keep their babies skin to skin. When I talk to parents though, they generally think skin-to-skin care is just about warmth and 'bonding'. On a deep, primitive level, babies are highly evolved to do everything in their power to stay in arms (where the bears can't get them!), preferably smooched up next to skin, and this is why they have a rooting reflex – sure it gets them to the food source, but babies root even when their tummies are full to bursting. Why? Because being at the breast automatically gives them skin to skin, which helps to regulate the breathing, heart rate, reflexes and temperature, at the same time as protecting them against infection and soothing their immature gut.[94]

The hEDS adult, it seems to me, is like a baby which has never grown up – their ANS continuing to misfire in spite of their maturity. Those with hEDS babies often remark on how their little one is even more dysregulated than their friends' non-hEDS babies. Whereas the non-hEDS baby will eventually start to thermoregulate, the hEDS baby can continue to struggle and the parents will have their work cut out seeing if baby is an 'always cold', 'always hot' or 'swings wildly' type of hEDSer and adjust the house thermostat accordingly. My grandson is an 'always hot' whilst his young sister was showing signs of Raynaud's before her first birthday. He runs around in a light t-shirt in mid-winter whilst she has her very own stash of microwaveable teddies! So it is with the breathing, swallowing, reflexes and so on – the hEDSer's ANS remains in full-on quirky mode past early infancy and will need the same degree of validation plus strategies as mum, particularly when they head out into the wider world.

If you imagine a 'squeaky scale' with the more settled baby near the lower end and the baby who can never be put down and hollers all evening even when rocked in arms up the higher end, then the hEDS baby can seem to fall off the top! Far from being caused by gas, reflux or over-indulgent parenting, the universal experience of babies being very upset and visibly sore in the evenings appears to be linked to circadian rhythms of various gut motility hormones and, of course, ensures close attention through the vulnerable hours of darkness in the fourth trimester.[95]

Colic is much more noticeable in the atopic baby,[96] so with the increased incidence of atopy in the hEDS population,[97] we shouldn't be surprised or alarmed if the hEDS baby is a squawker. As tempting as it is to suggest using colic drops or reflux medications, parents need reassurance that this is a normal, protective survival mechanism evolved over many thousands of years to keep babies safe and that babies who have close, responsive parenting are more likely to grow up secure and confident[98] – a proper happy ending if ever there was one!

*I'd take all of it again because it brought my baby girl safely into this world.*

Faye

# References

## CHAPTER 1

1   Malfait, F., Francomano, C., Byers, P., Belmont, J. *et al.* (2017). The 2017 international classification of the Ehlers-Danlos syndromes. *American Journal of Medical Genetics Part C: Seminars in Medical Genetics*, 175(1), pp.8–26.

2   Castori, M., Tinkle, B., Levy, H., Grahame, R., Malfait, F. and Hakim, A. (2017). A framework for the classification of joint hypermobility and related conditions. *American Journal of Medical Genetics Part C: Seminars in Medical Genetics*, 175(1), pp.148–157.

3   Demmler, J.C., Atkinson, M.D., Reinhold, E.J., Choy, E., Lyons, R.A. and Brophy, S.T. (2019). Diagnosed prevalence of Ehlers-Danlos syndrome and hypermobility spectrum disorder in Wales, UK: A national electronic cohort study and case-control comparison. *BMJ Open*, 9(11), e031365.

4   Ehlers-Danlos News (2020). Prevalence of EDS. Accessed on 01/04/2023 at https://ehlersdanlosnews.com/prevalence-of-eds.

5   Ricard-Blum, S. (2010). The collagen family. *Cold Spring Harbor Perspectives in Biology*, 3(1), a004978–a004978.

6   Di Lullo, G.A., Sweeney, S.M., Korkko, J., Ala-Kokko, L. and San Antonio, J.D. (2002). Mapping the ligand-binding sites and disease-associated mutations on the most abundant protein in the human, type 1 collagen. *Journal of Biological Chemistry*, 277(6), pp.4223–4231.

7   Shi, J.-W., Lai, Z.-Z., Yang, H.-L., Yang, S.-L. *et al.* (2020). Collagen at the maternal-fetal interface in human pregnancy. *International Journal of Biological Sciences*, 16(12), pp.2220–2234.

8   Levy, H.P. (2018). Hypermobile Ehlers-Danlos Syndrome. In M.P. Adam, G.M. Mirzaa, R.A. Pagon, S.E. Wallace *et al.* (eds) *GeneReviews®*. Accessed on 01/04/2023 at www.ncbi.nlm.nih.gov/books/NBK1279.

9   Malfait, F., Francomano, C., Byers, P., Belmont, J. *et al.* (2017). The 2017 international classification of the Ehlers-Danlos syndromes. *American Journal of Medical Genetics Part C: Seminars in Medical Genetics*, 175(1), pp.8–26.

10  Bowen, J.M., Sobey, G.J., Burrows, N.P., Colombi, M. *et al.* (2017). Ehlers-Danlos syndrome, classical type. *American Journal of Medical Genetics Part C: Seminars in Medical Genetics*, 175(1), pp.27–39.

11  Erdogan, F.G., Tufan, A., Guven, M., Goker, B. and Gurler, A. (2012). Association of hypermobility and ingrown nails. *Clinical Rheumatology*, 31(9), pp.1319–1322.

12  Edimo, C.O., Wajsberg, J.R., Wong, S., Nahmias, Z.P. and Riley, B.A. (2021). The dermatological aspects of hEDS in women. *International Journal of Women's Dermatology*. https://doi.org/10.1016/j.ijwd.2021.01.020.

13  Levy, H.P. (2018). Hypermobile Ehlers-Danlos Syndrome. In M.P. Adam, G.M. Mirzaa, R.A. Pagon, S.E. Wallace *et al.* (eds) *GeneReviews®*. Accessed on 01/04/2023 at www.ncbi.nlm.nih.gov/books/NBK1279.

14  Adib, N., Davies, K., Grahame, R., Woo, P. and Murray, K.J. (2005). Joint hypermobility syndrome in childhood. A not so benign multisystem disorder? *Rheumatology*, 44(6), pp.744–750.

## CHAPTER 2

1  Walker, J. (2020). Skeletal system 2: Structure and function of the musculoskeletal system. *Nursing Times*. Accessed on 01/04/2023 at www.nursingtimes.net/clinical-archive/orthopaedics/skeletal-system-2-structure-and-function-of-the-musculo-skeletal-system-24-02-2020.

2  Physiopedia. (2011). Beighton Score. Accessed on 01/04/2023 at www.physio-pedia.com/Beighton_score.

3  Meester, J.A.N., Verstraeten, A., Schepers, D., Alaerts, M., Van Laer, L. and Loeys, B.L. (2017). Differences in manifestations of Marfan syndrome, Ehlers-Danlos syndrome, and Loeys-Dietz syndrome. *Annals of Cardiothoracic Surgery*, 6(6), pp.582–594.

4  Munir, U., Mabrouk, A. and Morgan, S. (2021). Hallux varus. In *Statpearls*. Treasure Island, FL: Statpearl Publishing. Accessed on 01/04/2023 at www.ncbi.nlm.nih.gov/books/NBK470261.

5  Buryk-Iggers, S., Mittal, N., Santa Mina, D., Adams, S.C. *et al.* (2022). Exercise and rehabilitation in people with Ehlers-Danlos syndrome: A systematic review. *Archives of Rehabilitation Research and Clinical Translation*, 4(2), 100189.

6  Griffin Occupational Therapy (2018). Let's talk about proprioception – our hidden sixth sense! Accessed on 01/04/2023 at www.griffinot.com/what-is-proprioception.

7  Clayton, H.A., Jones, S.A.H. and Henriques, D.Y.P. (2015). Proprioceptive precision is impaired in Ehlers–Danlos syndrome. *SpringerPlus*. https://doi.org/10.1186/s40064-015-1089-1.

8  Hand, L. (2012). Connecting instability and ankle osteoarthritis. *Lower Extremity Review Magazine*. Accessed on 19/01/2023 at https://lermagazine.com/article/connecting-instability-and-ankle-osteoarthritis.

9  Broida, S.E., Sweeney, A.P., Gottschalk, M.B. and Wagner, E.R. (2021). Management of shoulder instability in hypermobility-type Ehlers-Danlos syndrome. *JSES Reviews, Reports, and Techniques*, 1(3), pp.155–164.

10  Betti, L. (2017). Human variation in pelvic shape and the effects of climate and past population history. *Anatomical Record*, 300(4), pp.687–697.

11  Wikipedia (2023). Pelvis. Accessed on 19/01/2023 at https://en.m.wikipedia.org/wiki/Pelvis.

12  Wu, W.H., Meijer, O.G., Uegaki, K., Mens, J.M.A. *et al.* (2004). Pregnancy-related pelvic girdle pain (PPP), I: Terminology, clinical presentation, and prevalence. *European Spine Journal*, 13(7), pp.575–589.

13  Ali, A., Andrzejowski, P., Kanakaris, N.K. and Giannoudis, P.V. (2020). Pelvic girdle pain, hypermobility spectrum disorder and hypermobility-type Ehlers-Danlos syndrome: A narrative literature review. *Journal of Clinical Medicine*, 9(12), 3992.

14  Aubry-Rozier, B., Schwitzguebel, A., Valerio, F., Tanniger, J. *et al.* (2021). Are patients with hypermobile Ehlers–Danlos syndrome or hypermobility spectrum disorder so different? *Rheumatology International*, 41(10), pp.1785–1794.

15  Aubry-Rozier, B., Schwitzguebel, A., Valerio, F., Tanniger, J. *et al.* (2021). Are patients with hypermobile Ehlers–Danlos syndrome or hypermobility spectrum disorder so different? *Rheumatology International*, 41(10), pp.1785–1794.

16  Mazziotti, G., Dordoni, C., Doga, M., Galderisi, F. *et al.* (2016). High prevalence of radiological vertebral fractures in adult patients with Ehlers–Danlos syndrome. *Bone*, 84, pp.88–92.

17  Inácio, P. (2020). Overlap symptoms of EDS, osteogenesis imperfecta may be new EDS type. Ehlers-Danlos News. Accessed on 19/01/2023 at https://ehlersdanlosnews.com/2020/01/23/overlap-symptoms-of-eds-and-osteogenesis-imperfecta-may-be-new-eds-type-researchers-contend.

18  Gazit, Y., Jacob, G. and Grahame, R. (2016). Ehlers–Danlos syndrome – hypermobility type: A much neglected multisystemic disorder. *Rambam Maimonides Medical Journal*, 7(4), e0034.

19  Berglund, B., Nordström, G., Hagberg, C. and Mattiasson, A.-C. (2005). Foot pain and disability in individuals with Ehlers–Danlos syndrome (EDS): Impact on daily life activities. *Disability and Rehabilitation*, 27(4), pp.164–169.

20  American Academy of Orthopaedic Surgeons (2022). Plantar Fasciitis and Bone Spurs. OrthoInfo. Accessed on 05/04/2023 at https://orthoinfo.aaos.org/en/diseases--conditions/plantar-fasciitis-and-bone-spurs.

21  American Academy of Orthopaedic Surgeons (2022). Morton's Neuroma. Accessed on 05/04/2023 at https://orthoinfo.aaos.org/en/diseases--conditions/mortons-neuroma.

## CHAPTER 3

1  Jarvis, S. and Saman, J.S. (2018). Cardiac system 1: Anatomy and physiology. *Nursing Times*. Accessed on 05/04/2023 at www.nursingtimes.net/clinical-archive/cardiovascular-clinical-archive/cardiac-system-1-anatomy-and-physiology-29-01-2018.

2  www.medi.de. (2020). Veins. Accessed on 05/04/2023 at www.medi.de/en/diagnosis-treatment/venous-disorders/anatomy-veins.

3  Gordan, R., Gwathmey, J.K. and Xie, L.-H. (2015). Autonomic and endocrine control of cardiovascular function. *World Journal of Cardiology*, 7(4), pp.204–214.

Guyenet, P.G. and Bayliss, D.A. (2015). Neural control of breathing and $CO_2$ homeostasis. *Neuron*, 87(5), pp.946–961.

4  Genetic and Rare Diseases Information Center (GARD) (2017). Vascular Ehlers-Danlos Syndrome. Accessed on 05/04/2023 at https://rarediseases.info.nih.gov/diseases/2082/vascular-ehlers-danlos-syndrome.

5  Camerota, F., Castori, M., Celletti, C., Colotto, M. *et al.* (2014). Heart rate, conduction and ultrasound abnormalities in adults with joint hypermobility syndrome/

Ehlers-Danlos syndrome, hypermobility type. *Clinical Rheumatology*, 33(7), pp.981–987.

6   Tinkle, B., Castori, M., Berglund, B., Cohen, H. *et al.* (2017). Hypermobile Ehlers-Danlos syndrome (a.k.a. Ehlers-Danlos syndrome type III and Ehlers-Danlos syndrome hypermobility type): Clinical description and natural history. *American Journal of Medical Genetics Part C: Seminars in Medical Genetics*, 175(1), pp.48–69.

7   Hakim, A., O'Callaghan, C., De Wandele, I., Stiles, L. *et al.* (2017). Cardiovascular autonomic dysfunction in Ehlers-Danlos syndrome – hypermobile type (for non-experts). Accessed on 19/01/2023 at www.ehlers-danlos.com/2017-eds-classification-non-experts/cardiovascular-autonomic-dysfunction-ehlers-danlos-syndrome-hypermobile-type.

Miller, A.J., Schubart, J.R., Sheehan, T., Bascom, R. and Francomano, C.A. (2020). Arterial elasticity in Ehlers-Danlos syndromes. *Genes*. https://doi.org/10.3390/genes11010055.

8   Morrison, J. (2017). Managing fatigue, sleeping problems and brain fog. Ehlers-Danlos Support UK. Accessed on 19/01/2023 at www.ehlers-danlos.org/information/managing-fatigue-sleeping-problems-and-brain-fog.

9   Gazit, Y., Nahir, A.M., Grahame, R. and Jacob, G. (2003). Dysautonomia in the joint hypermobility syndrome. *American Journal of Medicine*, 115(1), pp.33–40.

Castori, M. and Voermans, N.C. (2014). Neurological manifestations of Ehlers-Danlos syndrome(s): A review. *Iranian Journal of Neurology*, 13(4), pp.190–208.

10  Tasnim, S., Tang, C., Musini, V.M. and Wright, J.M. (2020). Effect of alcohol on blood pressure. *Cochrane Database of Systematic Reviews*. https://doi.org/10.1002/14651858.cd012787.pub2.

11  Hakim, A., O'Callaghan, C., De Wandele, I., Stiles, L., Pocinki, A. and Rowe, P. (2017). Cardiovascular autonomic dysfunction in Ehlers-Danlos syndrome – hypermobile type. *American Journal of Medical Genetics Part C: Seminars in Medical Genetics*, 175(1), pp.168–174.

12  Hecht, K., Vogt, W.F., Wachtel, E. and Fietze, I. (1991). Relationship between insomnia and arterial hypotension. *Pneumologie (Stuttgart, Germany)*, 45 Suppl. 1, pp.196–199.

13  Castori, M. (2012). Ehlers-Danlos syndrome, hypermobility type: An underdiagnosed hereditary connective tissue disorder with mucocutaneous, articular, and systemic manifestations. *ISRN Dermatology*. https://doi.org/10.5402/2012/751768.

14  Levy, H.P. (2018). Hypermobile Ehlers-Danlos Syndrome. In M.P. Adam, G.M. Mirzaa, R.A. Pagon, S.E. Wallace *et al.* (eds) *GeneReviews®*. Accessed on 05/04/2023 at www.ncbi.nlm.nih.gov/books/NBK1279.

15  Hugon-Rodin, J., Lebègue, G., Becourt, S., Hamonet, C. and Gompel, A. (2016). Gynecologic symptoms and the influence on reproductive life in 386 women with hypermobility type Ehlers-Danlos syndrome: A cohort study. *Orphanet Journal of Rare Diseases*. https://doi.org/10.1186/s13023-016-0511-2.

16  Paepe, A.D. and Malfait, F. (2004). Bleeding and bruising in patients with Ehlers-Danlos syndrome and other collagen vascular disorders. *British Journal of Haematology*, 127(5), pp.491–500.

17  Castori, M. (2012). Ehlers-Danlos syndrome, hypermobility type: An underdiagnosed hereditary connective tissue disorder with mucocutaneous, articular, and systemic manifestations. *ISRN Dermatology*. https://doi.org/10.5402/2012/751768.

18 Chaudhry, R. and Bordoni, B. (2019). Anatomy, thorax, lungs. In *Statpearls*. Treasure Island, FL: Statpearl Publishing. Accessed on 05/04/2023 at www.ncbi.nlm.nih.gov/books/NBK470197.

19 Chohan, K., Mittal, N., McGillis, L., Lopez-Hernandez, L. *et al.* (2021). A review of respiratory manifestations and their management in Ehlers-Danlos syndromes and hypermobility spectrum disorders. *Chronic Respiratory Disease*. https://doi.org/10.1177/14799731211025313.

20 Morgan, A.W., Pearson, S.B., Davies, S., Gooi, H.C. and Bird, H.A. (2007). Asthma and airways collapse in two heritable disorders of connective tissue. *Annals of the Rheumatic Diseases*, 66(10), pp.1369–1373.

21 Morgan, A.W., Pearson, S.B., Davies, S., Gooi, H.C. and Bird, H.A. (2007). Asthma and airways collapse in two heritable disorders of connective tissue. *Annals of the Rheumatic Diseases*, 66(10), pp.1369–1373.

## CHAPTER 4

1 WebMD Editorial Contributors (2022). Your digestive system. WebMD. Accessed on 05/04/2023 at www.webmd.com/heartburn-gerd/your-digestive-system.

2 National Cancer Institute (2019). General Structure of the Digestive System. SEER Training Module. Accessed on 05/04/2023 at https://training.seer.cancer.gov/anatomy/digestive/structure.html.

3 Ehlers-Danlos Support UK (2018). Gastrointestinal problems in hypermobile Ehlers-Danlos syndrome and hypermobility spectrum disorders. Accessed on 05/04/2023 at www.ehlers-danlos.org/information/gastrointestinal-problems-in-hypermobile-ehlers-danlos-syndrome-and-hypermobility-spectrum-disorders.

4 Fikree, A. and Byrne, P. (2021). Management of functional gastrointestinal disorders. *Clinical Medicine*, 21(1), pp.44–52.

5 Al-Rawi, Z.S. (2004). Joint mobility in people with hiatus hernia. *Rheumatology*, 43(5), pp.574–576.

6 Lam, C., Amarasinghe, G., Zarate-Lopez, N., Fikree, A. *et al.* (2022). Gastrointestinal symptoms and nutritional issues in patients with hypermobility disorders: Assessment, diagnosis and management. *Frontline Gastroenterology*. https://doi.org/10.1136/flgastro-2022-102088.

Nelson, A.D., Mouchli, M.A., Valentin, N., Deyle, D. *et al.* (2015). Ehlers Danlos syndrome and gastrointestinal manifestations: A 20-year experience at Mayo Clinic. *Neurogastroenterology and Motility*, 27(11), pp.1657–1666.

Alomari, M., Hitawala, A., Chadalavada, P., Covut, F. *et al.* (2020). Prevalence and predictors of gastrointestinal dysmotility in patients with hypermobile Ehlers-Danlos syndrome: A tertiary care center experience. *Cureus*. https://doi.org/10.7759/cureus.7881.

7 Lam, C., Amarasinghe, G., Zarate-Lopez, N., Fikree, A. *et al.* (2022). Gastrointestinal symptoms and nutritional issues in patients with hypermobility disorders: Assessment, diagnosis and management. *Frontline Gastroenterology*. https://doi.org/10.1136/flgastro-2022-102088.

Alomari, M., Hitawala, A., Chadalavada, P., Covut, F. *et al.* (2020). Prevalence and predictors of gastrointestinal dysmotility in patients with hypermobile Ehlers-Danlos syndrome: A tertiary care center experience. *Cureus.* https://doi.org/10.7759/cureus.7881.

8    Zeitoun, J.-D., Lefèvre, J.H., de Parades, V., Séjourné, C. *et al.* (2013). Functional digestive symptoms and quality of life in patients with Ehlers-Danlos syndromes: Results of a national cohort study on 134 patients. *PLoS ONE*, 8(11), p.e80321.

9    Choudhary, A., Fikree, A. and Aziz, Q. (2021). Overlap between irritable bowel syndrome and hypermobile Ehlers–Danlos syndrome: An unexplored clinical phenotype? *American Journal of Medical Genetics Part C: Seminars in Medical Genetics*, 187(4), pp.561–569.

10   Fikree, A., Chelimsky, G., Collins, H., Kovacic, K. and Aziz, Q. (2017). Gastrointestinal involvement in the Ehlers-Danlos syndromes. *American Journal of Medical Genetics Part C: Seminars in Medical Genetics*, 175(1), pp.181–187.

11   Kinsinger, S. (2017). Cognitive-behavioral therapy for patients with irritable bowel syndrome: Current insights. *Psychology Research and Behavior Management*, 10, pp.231–237.

12   TeachMe Anatomy (2018). The Peritoneum. Accessed on 05/04/2023 at https://teachmeanatomy.info/abdomen/areas/peritoneum.

13   Rezaie, A., Raphael, Y., Sukov, R. and Liu, X. (2018). Ehlers-Danlos syndrome type III (EDS) and visceroptosis: Getting to the bottom of this diagnosis: 469. *American Journal of Gastroenterology*, 113, pp.S270–S271.

     Takakura, W., Raphael, Y., Sukov, R. and Rezaie, A. (2020). S3153 Hypermobile Ehlers-Danlos syndrome and visceroptosis. *American Journal of Gastroenterology*, 115, pp.S1656–S1657.

14   Lammers, K., Lince, S.L., Spath, M.A., van Kempen, L.C.L.T. *et al.* (2011). Pelvic organ prolapse and collagen-associated disorders. *International Urogynecology Journal*, 23(3), pp.313–319.

15   Vighi, G., Marcucci, F., Sensi, L., Di Cara, G. and Frati, F. (2008). Allergy and the gastrointestinal system. *Clinical and Experimental Immunology*, 153, pp.3–6.

16   Brooks, R.S., Grady, J., Lowder, T.W. and Blitshteyn, S. (2021). Prevalence of gastrointestinal, cardiovascular, autonomic and allergic manifestations in hospitalized patients with Ehlers-Danlos syndrome: A case-control study. *Rheumatology.* https://doi.org/10.1093/rheumatology/keaa926.

     Seneviratne, S.L., Maitland, A. and Afrin, L. (2017). Mast cell disorders in Ehlers-Danlos syndrome. *American Journal of Medical Genetics Part C: Seminars in Medical Genetics*, 175(1), pp.226–236.

17   Larsen, J.N., Broge, L. and Jacobi, H. (2016). Allergy immunotherapy: The future of allergy treatment. *Drug Discovery Today*, 21(1), pp.26–37.

18   Krystel-Whittemore, M., Dileepan, K.N. and Wood, J.G. (2016). Mast cell: A multifunctional master cell. *Frontiers in Immunology*, 6, p.620.

19   Seneviratne, S.L., Maitland, A. and Afrin, L. (2017). Mast cell disorders in Ehlers-Danlos syndrome. *American Journal of Medical Genetics Part C: Seminars in Medical Genetics*, 175(1), pp.226–236.

     Brock, I., Prendergast, W. and Maitland, A. (2021). Mast cell activation disease and immunoglobulin deficiency in patients with hypermobile Ehlers-Danlos syndrome/hypermobility spectrum disorder. *American Journal of Medical Genetics Part C: Seminars in Medical Genetics*, 187(4), pp.473–481.

20  Schubart, J.R., Schaefer, E., Janicki, P., Adhikary, S.D. *et al.* (2019). Resistance to local anesthesia in people with the Ehlers-Danlos syndromes presenting for dental surgery. *Journal of Dental Anesthesia and Pain Medicine*, 19(5), pp.261–270.

Arendt-Nielsen, L., Kaalund, S., Bjerring, P. and Høgsaa, B. (1990). Insufficient effect of local analgesics in Ehlers Danlos type III patients (connective tissue disorder). *Acta Anaesthesiologica Scandinavica*, 34(5), pp.358–361.

21  Do, T., Diamond, S., Green, C. and Warren, M. (2021). Nutritional implications of patients with dysautonomia and hypermobility syndromes. *Current Nutrition Reports*, 10(4), pp.324–333.

## CHAPTER 5

1   National Institute on Deafness and Other Communication Disorders (2018). How Do We Hear? Accessed on 05/04/2023 at www.nidcd.nih.gov/health/how-do-we-hear.

2   Hearing Link Services (2018). How the Ear Works. Accessed on 05/04/2023 at www.hearinglink.org/your-hearing/about-hearing/how-the-ear-works.

3   Baguley, D., McFerran, D. and Hall, D. (2013). Tinnitus. *The Lancet*, 382(9904), pp.1600–1607.

4   Baguley, D., McFerran, D. and Hall, D. (2013). Tinnitus. *The Lancet*, 382(9904), pp.1600–1607.

5   Vielsmeier, V., Kleinjung, T., Strutz, J., Bürgers, R., Kreuzer, P.M. and Langguth, B. (2011). Tinnitus with temporomandibular joint disorders. *Otolaryngology–Head and Neck Surgery*, 145(5), pp.748–752.

6   George, L. and Wijeyesakere, S. (2004). The incidence of tinnitus in people with disorders of the temporomandibular joint. *International Tinnitus Journal*, 10(2), pp.174–176.

7   Mitakides, J. and Tinkle, B.T. (2017). Oral and mandibular manifestations in the Ehlers-Danlos syndromes. *American Journal of Medical Genetics Part C: Seminars in Medical Genetics*, 175(1), pp.220–225.

8   Silverstein, H., Smith, J. and Kellermeyer, B. (2019). Stapes hypermobility as a possible cause of hyperacusis. *American Journal of Otolaryngology*, 40(2), pp.247–252.

9   Tidy, C. (2021). Ehlers-Danlos syndrome. Patient. Accessed on 23/01/2023 at https://patient.info/bones-joints-muscles/ehlers-danlos-syndrome-leaflet.

Hear-it.org. (n.d.). Ehlers-Danlos Syndrome. Accessed on 23/01/2023 at www.hear-it.org/Ehlers-Danlos-Syndrome.

10  Rustom, I. (2022). Rapid response: Common drugs that cause tinnitus. *BMJ*. Accessed on 06/04/2023 at www.bmj.com/rapid-response/2011/10/31/common-drugs-cause-tinnitus.

11  Weir, F.W., Hatch, J.L., Muus, J.S., Wallace, S.A. and Meyer, T.A. (2016). Audiologic outcomes in Ehlers-Danlos syndrome. *Otology and Neurotology*, 37(6), pp.748–752.

12  Lomas, J., Gurgenci, T., Jackson, C. and Campbell, D. (2021). Temporomandibular dysfunction. *Australian Journal of General Practice*, 47(4), pp.212–215.

13  National Institute for Health and Care Excellence (NICE) (2021). Temporomandibular Disorders (TMDs). Accessed on 06/04/2023 at https://cks.nice.org.uk/topics/temporomandibular-disorders-tmds.

National Institute of Dental and Craniofacial Research (2018). Prevalence of TMJD and Its Signs and Symptoms. Accessed on 06/04/2023 at www.nidcr.nih.gov/research/data-statistics/facial-pain/prevalence.

14   Castori, M. and Voermans, N.C. (2014). Neurological manifestations of Ehlers-Danlos syndrome(s): A review. *Iranian Journal of Neurology*, 13(4), pp.190–208.

Harinstein, D., Buckingham, R.B., Braun, T., Oral, K. *et al.* (1988). Systemic joint laxity (the hypermobile joint syndrome) is associated with temporomandibular joint dysfunction. *Arthritis and Rheumatism*, 31(10), pp.1259–1264.

De Costa, P.J., Van den Berghe, L.I. and Martens, L.C. (2005) Generalized joint hypermobility and temporomandibular disorders: Inherited connective tissue disease as a model with maximum expression. *Journal of Orofacial Pain*, 19(1), pp.47–57.

15   Mitakides, J. and Tinkle, B.T. (2017). Oral and mandibular manifestations in the Ehlers-Danlos syndromes. *American Journal of Medical Genetics Part C: Seminars in Medical Genetics*, 175(1), pp.220–225.

16   Wikipedia (2023). Human Nose. Accessed on 24/01/2023 at https://en.m.wikipedia.org/wiki/Human_nose.

17   Gaisl, T., Giunta, C., Bratton, D.J., Sutherland, K. *et al.* (2017). Obstructive sleep apnoea and quality of life in Ehlers-Danlos syndrome: A parallel cohort study. *Thorax*, 72(8), pp.729–735.

18   Levy, H.P. (2018). Hypermobile Ehlers-Danlos Syndrome. In M.P. Adam, G.M. Mirzaa, R.A. Pagon, S.E. Wallace *et al.* (eds) *GeneReviews®*. Accessed on 06/04/2023 at www.ncbi.nlm.nih.gov/books/NBK1279.

19   Van Camp, N., Aerden, T. and Politis, C. (2020). Problems in the orofacial region associated with Ehlers-Danlos and Marfan syndromes: A case series. *British Journal of Oral and Maxillofacial Surgery*, 58(2), pp.208–213.

20   Hanisch, M., Blanck-Lubarsch, M., Bohner, L., Suwelack, D., Kleinheinz, J. and Köppe, J. (2020). Oral conditions and oral health-related quality of life of people with Ehlers-Danlos syndromes (EDS): A questionnaire-based cross-sectional study. *Medicina*. https://doi.org/10.3390/medicina56090448.

21   Celletti, C., Castori, M., La Torre, G., Grammatico, P., Morico, G. and Camerota, F. (2011). Reassessment of oral frenula in Ehlers-Danlos syndrome: A study of 32 patients with the hypermobility type. *American Journal of Medical Genetics Part A*, 155(12), pp.3157–3159.

22   Castori, M., Dordoni, C., Morlino, S., Sperduti, I. *et al.* (2015). Spectrum of mucocutaneous manifestations in 277 patients with joint hypermobility syndrome/Ehlers-Danlos syndrome, hypermobility type. *American Journal of Medical Genetics Part C: Seminars in Medical Genetics*, 169(1), pp.43–53.

23   Hunter, A. (2017). Speech, language, voice and swallowing in the Ehlers-Danlos syndromes. Ehlers-Danlos Support UK. Accessed on 06/04/2023 at www.ehlers-danlos.org/information/speech-language-voice-and-swallowing-in-the-ehlers-danlos-syndromes.

24   Birchall, M.A., Lam, C.M. and Wood, G. (2021). Throat and voice problems in Ehlers–Danlos syndromes and hypermobility spectrum disorders. *American Journal of Medical Genetics Part C: Seminars in Medical Genetics*, 187(4), pp.527–532.

## CHAPTER 6

1 Chawla, J. (2021). Central nervous system anatomy: Overview. eMedicine. Accessed on 06/04/2023 at https://emedicine.medscape.com/article/1948665-overview#a2.

2 Chawla, J. (2022). Peripheral nervous system anatomy. eMedicine. Accessed on 24/01/2023 at https://emedicine.medscape.com/article/1948687-overview?reg=1.

3 Markowsky, G. (2019). Physiology. Britannica. Accessed on 06/04/2023 at www.britannica.com/science/information-theory/Physiology.

4 Levy, A.R., Nnam, M., Gudesblatt, M. and Riley, B. (2020). An investigation of headaches in hypermobile Ehlers-Danlos syndrome. *Annals of Psychiatry and Clinical Neuroscience*, 3(3), 1034.

5 Bendik, E.M., Tinkle, B.T., Al-shuik, E., Levin, L. *et al.* (2011). Joint hypermobility syndrome: A common clinical disorder associated with migraine in women. *Cephalalgia*, 31(5), pp.603–613.

6 Henderson, F.C. (2016). Cranio-cervical instability in patients with hypermobility connective disorders. *Journal of Spine*. https://doi.org/10.4172/2165-7939.1000299.

7 Henderson, F.C., Austin, C., Benzel, E., Bolognese, P. *et al.* (2017). Neurological and spinal manifestations of the Ehlers-Danlos syndromes. *American Journal of Medical Genetics Part C: Seminars in Medical Genetics*, 175(1), pp.195–211.

8 Bendik, E.M., Tinkle, B.T., Al-shuik, E., Levin, L. *et al.* (2011). Joint hypermobility syndrome: A common clinical disorder associated with migraine in women. *Cephalalgia*, 31(5), pp.603–613.

9 Henderson, F.C., Austin, C., Benzel, E., Bolognese, P. *et al.* (2017). Neurological and spinal manifestations of the Ehlers-Danlos syndromes. *American Journal of Medical Genetics Part C: Seminars in Medical Genetics*, 175(1), pp.195–211.

10 Hiremath, S.B., Fitsiori, A., Boto, J., Torres, C. *et al.* (2020). The perplexity surrounding Chiari malformations – are we any wiser now? *American Journal of Neuroradiology*, 41(11), pp.1975–1981.

11 National Organization for Rare Disorders (NORD) (2014). Chiari Malformations. Accessed on 27/01/2023 at https://rarediseases.org/rare-diseases/chiari-malformations/?filter=ovr-ds-resources.

12 National Organization for Rare Disorders (NORD) (2014). Chiari Malformations. Accessed on 27/01/2023 at https://rarediseases.org/rare-diseases/chiari-malformations/?filter=ovr-ds-resources.

13 Klinge, P.M., Srivastava, V., McElroy, A., Leary, O.P. *et al.* (2022). Diseased filum terminale as a cause of tethered cord syndrome in Ehlers-Danlos syndrome: Histopathology, biomechanics, clinical presentation, and outcome of filum excision. *World Neurosurgery*, 162, pp.e492–e502.

14 Donnally III, C.J., Hanna, A. and Varacallo, M. (2020). Lumbar degenerative disk disease. In *Statpearls*. Treasure Island, FL: Statpearl Publishing. Accessed on 06/04/2023 at www.ncbi.nlm.nih.gov/books/NBK448134.

15 Wang, Y.-X.J., Griffith, J.F., Zeng, X.-J., Deng, M. *et al.* (2013). Prevalence and sex difference of lumbar disc space narrowing in elderly Chinese men and women: Osteoporotic fractures in men (Hong Kong) and osteoporotic fractures in women (Hong Kong) studies. *Arthritis and Rheumatism*, 65(4), pp.1004–1010.

16  Henderson, F.C., Austin, C., Benzel, E., Bolognese, P. *et al.* (2017). Neurological and spinal manifestations of the Ehlers-Danlos syndromes. *American Journal of Medical Genetics Part C: Seminars in Medical Genetics*, 175(1), pp.195–211.

17  Castori, M., Morlino, S., Celletti, C., Ghibellini, G. *et al.* (2013). Re-writing the natural history of pain and related symptoms in the joint hypermobility syndrome/ Ehlers-Danlos syndrome, hypermobility type. *American Journal of Medical Genetics Part A*, 161(12), pp.2989–3004.

18  Hakim, A. (2018). Fibromyalgia and chronic fatigue. Ehlers-Danlos Support UK. Accessed on 06/04/2023 at www.ehlers-danlos.org/information/ fibromyalgia-and-chronic-fatigue.

## CHAPTER 7

1   Wikipedia (2023). Urinary System. Accessed on 06/04/2023 at https://en.m.wikipedia.org/wiki/Urinary_system.

2   Sam, P., Jiang, J. and LaGrange, C.A. (2022). Anatomy, abdomen and pelvis, sphincter urethrae. In *Statpearls*. Treasure Island, FL: Statpearl Publishing. Accessed on 06/04/2023 at https://pubmed.ncbi.nlm.nih.gov/29494045.

3   Botlero, R., Urquhart, D.M., Davis, S.R. and Bell, R.J. (2008). Prevalence and incidence of urinary incontinence in women: Review of the literature and investigation of methodological issues. *International Journal of Urology*, 15(3), pp.230–234.

4   Thomas, T., Plymat, K., Blannin, J. and Meade, T. (1980). Prevalence of urinary incontinence. *BMJ*, 281. Accessed on 27/01/2023 at www.ncbi.nlm.nih.gov/pmc/ articles/PMC1714689/pdf/brmedj00046-0017.pdf.

5   Arunkalaivanan, A.S., Morrison, A., Jha, S. and Blann, A. (2009). Prevalence of urinary and faecal incontinence among female members of the Hypermobility Syndrome Association (HMSA). *Journal of Obstetrics and Gynaecology*, 29(2), pp.126–128.

6   Keane, D.P., Sims, T.J., Abrams, P. and Bailey, A.J. (1997). Analysis of collagen status in premenopausal nulliparous women with genuine stress incontinence. *British Journal of Obstetrics and Gynaecology*, 104(9), pp.994–998.

7   Mastoroudes, H., Giarenis, I., Cardozo, L., Srikrishna, S. *et al.* (2013). Lower urinary tract symptoms in women with benign joint hypermobility syndrome: A case-control study. *International Urogynecology Journal*, 24(9), pp.1553–1558.

8   Khullar, V. (2014) The bladder and EDS [Video file]. Ehlers-Danlos Support UK. Accessed on 06/04/2023 at www.ehlers-danlos.org/information/ video-the-bladder-and-eds.

9   Khullar, L., Morris, E., McHayle, A., Tailor, V.K. *et al.* (2019). Urinalysis is not a good test for urine tract infection in women with hypermobile EDS. Accessed on 27/01/2023 at www.ics.org/Abstracts/Publish/484/eposter/596.pdf.

10  Khullar, V. (2014) The bladder and EDS [Video file]. Ehlers-Danlos Support UK. Accessed on 06/04/2023 at www.ehlers-danlos.org/information/ video-the-bladder-and-eds.

11  Gilliam, E., Hoffman, J.D. and Yeh, G. (2020). Urogenital and pelvic complications in the Ehlers-Danlos syndromes and associated hypermobility spectrum disorders: A scoping review. *Clinical Genetics*, 97(1), pp.168–178.

12  Hugon-Rodin, J., Lebègue, G., Becourt, S., Hamonet, C. and Gompel, A. (2016). Gynecologic symptoms and the influence on reproductive life in 386 women with hypermobility type Ehlers-Danlos syndrome: A cohort study. *Orphanet Journal of Rare Diseases*. https://doi.org/10.1186/s13023-016-0511-2.

13  Hugon-Rodin, J., Lebègue, G., Becourt, S., Hamonet, C. and Gompel, A. (2016). Gynecologic symptoms and the influence on reproductive life in 386 women with hypermobility type Ehlers-Danlos syndrome: A cohort study. *Orphanet Journal of Rare Diseases*. https://doi.org/10.1186/s13023-016-0511-2.

14  El-Hemaidi, I., Gharaibeh, A. and Shehata, H. (2007). Menorrhagia and bleeding disorders. *Current Opinion in Obstetrics and Gynecology*, 19(6), pp.513–520.

15  National Institute for Health and Care Excellence (NICE) (2021). CKS is only available in the UK. Accessed on 06/04/2023 at https://cks.nice.org.uk/topics/ temporomandibular-disorders-tmds.

16  Hugon-Rodin, J., Lebègue, G., Becourt, S., Hamonet, C. and Gompel, A. (2016). Gynecologic symptoms and the influence on reproductive life in 386 women with hypermobility type Ehlers-Danlos syndrome: A cohort study. *Orphanet Journal of Rare Diseases*. https://doi.org/10.1186/s13023-016-0511-2.

17  Hugon-Rodin, J., Lebègue, G., Becourt, S., Hamonet, C. and Gompel, A. (2016). Gynecologic symptoms and the influence on reproductive life in 386 women with hypermobility type Ehlers-Danlos syndrome: A cohort study. *Orphanet Journal of Rare Diseases*. https://doi.org/10.1186/s13023-016-0511-2.

18  Gilliam, E., Hoffman, J.D. and Yeh, G. (2020). Urogenital and pelvic complications in the Ehlers-Danlos syndromes and associated hypermobility spectrum disorders: A scoping review. *Clinical Genetics*, 97(1), pp.168–178.

Al-Rawi, Z.S. and Al-Rawi, Z.T. (1982). Joint hypermobility in women with genital prolapse. *The Lancet*, 319(8287), pp.1439–1441.

Aydeniz, A., Dikensoy, E., Cebesoy, B., Altindağ, O., Gürsoy, S. and Balat, O. (2010). The relation between genitourinary prolapse and joint hypermobility in Turkish women. *Archives of Gynecology and Obstetrics*, 281(2), pp.301–304.

19  Tommy's (2023). Miscarriage Statistics. Accessed on 06/04/2023 at www. tommys.org/baby-loss-support/miscarriage-information-and-support/ miscarriage-statistics#general.

20  El-Hemaidi, I., Gharaibeh, A. and Shehata, H. (2007). Menorrhagia and bleeding disorders. *Current Opinion in Obstetrics and Gynecology*, 19(6), pp.513–520.

Lind, J. and Wallenburg, H.C.S. (2002). Pregnancy and the Ehlers-Danlos syndrome: A retrospective study in a Dutch population. *Acta Obstetricia et Gynecologica Scandinavica*, 81(4), pp.293–300.

21  El-Hemaidi, I., Gharaibeh, A. and Shehata, H. (2007). Menorrhagia and bleeding disorders. *Current Opinion in Obstetrics and Gynecology*, 19(6), pp.513–520.

Lind, J. and Wallenburg, H.C.S. (2002). Pregnancy and the Ehlers-Danlos syndrome: A retrospective study in a Dutch population. *Acta Obstetricia et Gynecologica Scandinavica*, 81(4), pp.293–300.

22  Tommy's (2023). Miscarriage Statistics. Accessed on 06/04/2023 at www. tommys.org/baby-loss-support/miscarriage-information-and-support/ miscarriage-statistics#general.

23   Sundelin, H.E.K., Stephansson, O., Johansson, K. and Ludvigsson, J.F. (2016). Pregnancy outcome in joint hypermobility syndrome and Ehlers-Danlos syndrome. *Acta Obstetricia et Gynecologica Scandinavica*, 96(1), pp.114–119.

Lind, J. and Wallenburg, H.C.S. (2002). Pregnancy and the Ehlers-Danlos syndrome: A retrospective study in a Dutch population. *Acta Obstetricia et Gynecologica Scandinavica*, 81(4), pp.293–300.

24   Hugon-Rodin, J., Lebègue, G., Becourt, S., Hamonet, C. and Gompel, A. (2016). Gynecologic symptoms and the influence on reproductive life in 386 women with hypermobility type Ehlers-Danlos syndrome: A cohort study. *Orphanet Journal of Rare Diseases*. https://doi.org/10.1186/s13023-016-0511-2.

Sundelin, H.E.K., Stephansson, O., Johansson, K. and Ludvigsson, J.F. (2016). Pregnancy outcome in joint hypermobility syndrome and Ehlers-Danlos syndrome. *Acta Obstetricia et Gynecologica Scandinavica*, 96(1), pp.114–119.

Lind, J. and Wallenburg, H.C.S. (2002). Pregnancy and the Ehlers-Danlos syndrome: A retrospective study in a Dutch population. *Acta Obstetricia et Gynecologica Scandinavica*, 81(4), pp.293–300.

## CHAPTER 8

1   Wikipedia (2023). Autonomic Nervous System. Accessed on 06/04/2023 at https://en.m.wikipedia.org/wiki/Autonomic_nervous_system.

2   Grigoriou, E., Boris, J.R. and Dormans, J.P. (2015). Postural orthostatic tachycardia syndrome (POTS): Association with Ehlers-Danlos syndrome and orthopaedic considerations. *Clinical Orthopaedics and Related Research*, 473(2), pp.722–728.

Kanjwal, K., Saeed, B., Karabin, B., Kanjwal, Y. and Grubb, B.P. (2010). Comparative clinical profile of postural orthostatic tachycardia patients with and without joint hypermobility syndrome. *Indian Pacing and Electrophysiology Journal*, 10(4), pp.173–178.

3   Gazit, Y., Nahir, A.M., Grahame, R. and Jacob, G. (2003). Dysautonomia in the joint hypermobility syndrome. *American Journal of Medicine*, 115(1), pp.33–40.

4   Raj, S.R. (2018). Autonomic dysfunction and EDS: An introduction. Ehlers-Danlos Society. Accessed on 30/01/2023 at https://youtu.be/zTndxPRJ9N8.

5   Schondorf, R. and Low, P.A. (1993). Idiopathic postural orthostatic tachycardia syndrome. *Neurology*, 43(1 Part 1), pp.132–137.

6   Freeman, R., Wieling, W., Axelrod, F.B., Benditt, D.G. *et al.* (2011). Consensus statement on the definition of orthostatic hypotension, neurally mediated syncope and the postural tachycardia syndrome. *Autonomic Neuroscience*, 161(1–2), pp.46–48.

7   Pocinki, A. (2017). Evaluation and management of autonomic dysfunction in EDS [Video file]. Ehlers-Danlos Society. Accessed on 30/01/2023 at https://youtu.be/6pmv_Pt2ulY.

8   Raj, S.R. (2018). Autonomic dysfunction and EDS: An introduction [Video file]. Ehlers-Danlos Society. Accessed on 30/01/2023 at https://youtu.be/zTndxPRJ9N8.

9   Stephenson, L.A. and Kolka, M.A. (1993). Thermoregulation in women. *Exercise and Sport Sciences Reviews*, 21, pp.231–262.

10   Pocinki, A. (2017). Evaluation and management of autonomic dysfunction in EDS [Video file]. Ehlers-Danlos Society. Accessed on 30/01/2023 at https://youtu.be/6pmv_Pt2ulY.

11   Hakim, A., O'Callaghan, C., De Wandele, l., Stiles, L., Pocinki, A. and Rowe, P. (2017). Cardiovascular autonomic dysfunction in Ehlers-Danlos syndrome – hypermobile type. *American Journal of Medical Genetics Part C: Seminars in Medical Genetics*, 175(1), pp.168–174.

12   Gordan, R., Gwathmey, J.K. and Xie, L.-H. (2015). Autonomic and endocrine control of cardiovascular function. *World Journal of Cardiology*, 7(4), pp.204–214.

13   Hecht, K., Vogt, W.F., Wachtel, E. and Fietze, l. (1991). Relationship between insomnia and arterial hypotension. *Pneumologie (Stuttgart, Germany)*, 45 Suppl. 1, pp.196–199.

14   Hamonet, C., Delarue, M., Lefevre, J., Rottembourg, J. and Zeitoun, J. (2021). Ehlers-Danlos syndrome (EDS) : A common and often disregarded cause of serious gastrointestinal complications in children and adults. *Scholarly Journal of Otolaryngology*. https://doi.org/10.32474/SJO.2021.07.000256.

15   Pocinki, A. (2017). Evaluation and management of autonomic dysfunction in EDS [Video file]. Ehlers-Danlos Society. Accessed on 30/01/2023 at https://youtu.be/6pmv_Pt2ulY.

16   Hunter, A. (2017). Speech, language, voice and swallowing in the Ehlers-Danlos syndromes. Ehlers-Danlos Support UK. Accessed on 06/04/2023 at www.ehlers-danlos.org/information/speech-language-voice-and-swallowing-in-the-ehlers-danlos-syndromes.

17   Hakim, A., De Wandele, I., O'Callaghan, C., Pocinki, A. and Rowe, P. (2017). Chronic fatigue in Ehlers-Danlos syndrome – hypermobile type. *American Journal of Medical Genetics Part C: Seminars in Medical Genetics*, 175(1), pp.175–180.

18   Pocinki, A. (2019). Sleep disorders in Ehlers-Danlos and related syndromes: A panoply of paradoxes [Video file]. Accessed on 30/01/2023 at https://youtu.be/Tr6lv8_NVOw.

19   Morrison, J. (2017) Managing fatigue, sleeping problems and brain fog. Ehlers-Danlos Support UK. Accessed on 06/04/2023 at www.ehlers-danlos.org/information/managing-fatigue-sleeping-problems-and-brain-fog.

20   Arnold, A. (2016). Cognitive dysfunction and 'brain fog' in POTS. The Dysautonomia Dispatch. Accessed on 30/01/2023 at https://dysautonomiainternational.org/blog/wordpress/cognitive-dysfunction-and-brain-fog-in-pots.

21   Martín-Santos, R., Bulbena, A., Porta, M., Gago, J., Molina, L. and Duró, J.C. (1998). Association between joint hypermobility syndrome and panic disorder. *American Journal of Psychiatry*, 155(11), pp.1578–1583.

      Murray, B., Yashar, B.M., Uhlmann, W.R., Clauw, D.J. and Petty, E.M. (2013). Ehlers-Danlos syndrome, hypermobility type: A characterization of the patients' lived experience. *American Journal of Medical Genetics Part A*, 161(12), pp.2981–2988.

22   Pocinki, A. (2016). Webinar: 'Psychiatric misdiagnoses in EDS: When is anxiety not anxiety?' [Video file]. EDS Awareness. Accessed on 11/04/2023 at www.chronicpainpartners.com/webinar/free-webinar-psychiatric-misdiagnoses-eds-anxiety-not-anxiety.

      Kesserwani, H. (2020). Postural orthostatic tachycardia syndrome misdiagnosed as anxiety: A case report with a review of therapy and pathophysiology. *Cureus*. https://doi.org/10.7759/cureus.10881.

23  Pocinki, A. (2016). Webinar: 'Psychiatric misdiagnoses in EDS: When is anxiety not anxiety?' [Video file]. EDS Awareness. Accessed on 11/04/2023 at www.chronicpainpartners.com/webinar/free-webinar-psychiatric-misdiagnoses-eds-anxiety-not-anxiety.

Kesserwani, H. (2020). Postural orthostatic tachycardia syndrome misdiagnosed as anxiety: A case report with a review of therapy and pathophysiology. *Cureus.* https://doi.org/10.7759/cureus.10881.

24  Pocinki, A. (2016). Webinar: 'Psychiatric misdiagnoses in EDS: When is anxiety not anxiety?' [Video file]. EDS Awareness. Accessed on 11/04/2023 at www.chronicpainpartners.com/webinar/free-webinar-psychiatric-misdiagnoses-eds-anxiety-not-anxiety.

25  De Baets, S., De Temmerman, M., Calders, P., Malfait, F. *et al.* (2022). The impact of hypermobile 'Ehlers-Danlos Syndrome' and hypermobile spectrum disorder on interpersonal interactions and relationships. *Frontiers in Rehabilitation Sciences.* https://doi.org/10.3389/fresc.2022.832806.

## CHAPTER 9

1  Lind, J. and Wallenburg, H.C.S. (2002). Pregnancy and the Ehlers-Danlos syndrome: A retrospective study in a Dutch population. *Acta Obstetricia et Gynecologica Scandinavica*, 81(4), pp.293–300.

Sundelin, H.E.K., Stephansson, O., Johansson, K. and Ludvigsson, J.F. (2016). Pregnancy outcome in joint hypermobility syndrome and Ehlers-Danlos syndrome. *Acta Obstetricia et Gynecologica Scandinavica*, 96(1), pp.114–119.

2  National Institute for Health and Care Excellence (NICE) (2022). Intrapartum Care for Healthy Women and Babies: 1.1 Place of Birth. CG190. Accessed on 11/04/2023 at www.nice.org.uk/guidance/cg190/chapter/Recommendations#place-of-birth.

3  Sundelin, H.E.K., Stephansson, O., Johansson, K. and Ludvigsson, J.F. (2016). Pregnancy outcome in joint hypermobility syndrome and Ehlers-Danlos syndrome. *Acta Obstetricia et Gynecologica Scandinavica*, 96(1), pp.114–119.

4  Gruber, K.J., Cupito, S.H. and Dobson, C.F. (2013). Impact of doulas on healthy birth outcomes. *Journal of Perinatal Education*, 22(1), pp.49–58.

5  The King's Fund. (2023). *Reconfiguring Maternity Services.* Accessed on 11/04/2023 at www.kingsfund.org.uk/publications/reconfiguration-clinical-services/maternity-services.

6  National Institute for Health and Care Excellence (NICE) (2022). Intrapartum Care for Healthy Women and Babies: 1.1 Place of Birth. CG190. Accessed on 11/04/2023 at www.nice.org.uk/guidance/cg190/chapter/Recommendations#place-of-birth.

7  Castori, M., Morlino, S., Dordoni, C., Celletti, C. *et al.* (2012). Gynecologic and obstetric implications of the joint hypermobility syndrome (a.k.a. Ehlers-Danlos syndrome hypermobility type) in 82 Italian patients. *American Journal of Medical Genetics Part A*, 158A(9), pp.2176–2182.

8  Sundelin, H.E.K., Stephansson, O., Johansson, K. and Ludvigsson, J.F. (2016). Pregnancy outcome in joint hypermobility syndrome and Ehlers-Danlos syndrome. *Acta Obstetricia et Gynecologica Scandinavica*, 96(1), pp.114–119.

9   Nursing and Midwifery Council (2018). *The Code: Professional Standards of Practice and Behaviour for Nurses, Midwives and Nursing Associates*. London: Nursing and Midwifery Council. Accessed on 11/04/2023 at www.nmc.org.uk/globalassets/site-documents/nmc-publications/nmc-code.pdf.

10  Macfarlane, A., Blondel, B., Mohangoo, A., Cuttini, M., Nijhuis, J. *et al.* (2015). Wide differences in mode of delivery within Europe: Risk-stratified analyses of aggregated routine data from the Euro-Peristat study. *BJOG: International Journal of Obstetrics and Gynaecology*, 123(4), pp.559–568.

Statista (2023). Method of childbirth delivery in England 2022. Accessed on 11/04/2023 at www.statista.com/statistics/407706/method-of-delivery-in-england.

11  Lothian, J.A. (2014). Healthy birth practice #4: Avoid interventions unless they are medically necessary. *Journal of Perinatal Education*, 23(4), pp.198–206.

12  Schubart, J.R., Schaefer, E., Janicki, P., Adhikary, S.D. *et al.* (2019). Resistance to local anesthesia in people with the Ehlers-Danlos syndromes presenting for dental surgery. *Journal of Dental Anesthesia and Pain Medicine*, 19(5), pp.261–270.

Arendt-Nielsen, L., Kaalund, S., Bjerring, P. and Høgsaa, B. (1990). Insufficient effect of local analgesics in Ehlers Danlos type III patients (connective tissue disorder). *Acta Anaesthesiologica Scandinavica*, 34(5), pp.358–361.

13  Grigoriou, E., Boris, J.R. and Dormans, J.P. (2015). Postural orthostatic tachycardia syndrome (POTS): Association with Ehlers-Danlos syndrome and orthopaedic considerations. *Clinical Orthopaedics and Related Research*, 473(2), pp.722–728.

Kanjwal, K., Saeed, B., Karabin, B., Kanjwal, Y. and Grubb, B.P. (2010). Comparative clinical profile of postural orthostatic tachycardia patients with and without joint hypermobility syndrome. *Indian Pacing and Electrophysiology Journal*, 10(4), pp.173–178.

Gazit, Y., Nahir, A.M., Grahame, R. and Jacob, G. (2003). Dysautonomia in the joint hypermobility syndrome. *American Journal of Medicine*, 115(1), pp.33–40.

14  Seneviratne, S.L., Maitland, A. and Afrin, L. (2017). Mast cell disorders in Ehlers-Danlos syndrome. *American Journal of Medical Genetics Part C: Seminars in Medical Genetics*, 175(1), pp.226–236.

15  De Costa, P.J., Van den Berghe, L.I. and Martens, L.C. (2005) Generalized joint hypermobility and temporomandibular disorders: Inherited connective tissue disease as a model with maximum expression. *Journal of Orofacial Pain*, 19(1) pp 47–57.

16  Ali, A., Andrzejowski, P., Kanakaris, N.K. and Giannoudis, P.V. (2020). Pelvic girdle pain, hypermobility spectrum disorder and hypermobility-type Ehlers-Danlos syndrome: A narrative literature review. *Journal of Clinical Medicine*, 9(12), 3992.

17  Ahlqvist, K., Bjelland, E.K., Pingel, R., Schlager, A., Nilsson-Wikmar, L. and Kristiansson, P. (2020). The association of self-reported generalized joint hypermobility with pelvic girdle pain during pregnancy: A retrospective cohort study. *BMC Musculoskeletal Disorders.* https://doi.org/10.1186/s12891-020-03486-w..

18  Seneviratne, S.L., Maitland, A. and Afrin, L. (2017). Mast cell disorders in Ehlers-Danlos syndrome. *American Journal of Medical Genetics Part C: Seminars in Medical Genetics*, 175(1), pp.226–236.

19  Vora, R., Gupta, R., Mehta, M., Chaudhari, A., Pilani, A. and Patel, N. (2014). Pregnancy and skin. *Journal of Family Medicine and Primary Care*, 3(4), pp.318–324.

20  Wessling-Resnick, M. (2010). Iron homeostasis and the inflammatory response. *Annual Review of Nutrition*, 30(1), pp.105–122.

21  Soppi, E.T. (2018). Iron deficiency without anemia – a clinical challenge. *Clinical Case Reports*, 6(6), pp.1082–1086.

22  Achebe, M.M. and Gafter-Gvili, A. (2016). How I treat anemia in pregnancy: Iron, cobalamin, and folate. *Blood*, 129(8), pp.940–949.

23  Pavord, S., Myers, B., Robinson, S., Allard, S., Strong, J. and Oppenheimer, C. (2012). UK guidelines on the management of iron deficiency in pregnancy. *British Journal of Haematology*, 156(5), pp.588–600.

24  Miller, A.J., Schubart, J.R., Sheehan, T., Bascom, R. and Francomano, C.A. (2020). Arterial elasticity in Ehlers-Danlos syndromes. *Genes*, 11(1), p.55.

25  Wu, M., Chen, S.-W. and Jiang, S.-Y. (2015). Relationship between gingival inflammation and pregnancy. *Mediators of Inflammation*, 2015, pp.1–11.

26  Castori, M. (2012). Ehlers-Danlos syndrome, hypermobility type: An underdiagnosed hereditary connective tissue disorder with mucocutaneous, articular, and systemic manifestations. *ISRN Dermatology*. https://doi.org/10.5402/2012/751768.

27  Schubart, J.R., Schaefer, E., Janicki, P., Adhikary, S.D. *et al.* (2019). Resistance to local anesthesia in people with the Ehlers-Danlos syndromes presenting for dental surgery. *Journal of Dental Anesthesia and Pain Medicine*, 19(5), pp.261–270.

28  Do, T., Diamond, S., Green, C. and Warren, M. (2021). Nutritional implications of patients with dysautonomia and hypermobility syndromes. *Current Nutrition Reports*, 10(4), pp.324–333.

29  DePhillipo, N.N., Aman, Z.S., Kennedy, M.I., Begley, J.P., Moatshe, G. and LaPrade, R.F. (2018). Efficacy of vitamin C supplementation on collagen synthesis and oxidative stress after musculoskeletal injuries: A systematic review. *Orthopaedic Journal of Sports Medicine*, 6(10), 2325967118804454.

30  Piccioni, M.G., Derme, M., Salerno, L., Morrocchi, E. *et al.* (2019). Management of severe epistaxis during pregnancy: A case report and review of the literature. *Case Reports in Obstetrics and Gynecology*, 2019, pp.1–3.

31  Castori, M. (2012). Ehlers-Danlos syndrome, hypermobility type: An underdiagnosed hereditary connective tissue disorder with mucocutaneous, articular, and systemic manifestations. *ISRN Dermatology*. https://doi.org/10.5402/2012/751768.

32  Karthikeyan, A. and Venkat-Raman, N. (2018). Hypermobile Ehlers–Danlos syndrome and pregnancy. *Obstetric Medicine*, 11(3), pp.104–109.

33  Buryk-Iggers, S., Mittal, N., Santa Mina, D., Adams, S.C. *et al.* (2022). Exercise and rehabilitation in people with Ehlers-Danlos syndrome: A systematic review. *Archives of Rehabilitation Research and Clinical Translation*, 4(2), 100189.

34  Fu, Q. and Levine, B.D. (2015). Exercise in the postural orthostatic tachycardia syndrome. *Autonomic Neuroscience: Basic and Clinical*, 188, pp.86–89.

    Blitshteyn, S., Poya, H. and Bett, G.C.L. (2012). Pregnancy in postural tachycardia syndrome: Clinical course and maternal and fetal outcomes. *Journal of Maternal-Fetal and Neonatal Medicine*, 25(9), pp.1631–1634.

35  Negro, A., Delaruelle, Z., Ivanova, T.A., Khan, S. *et al.* (2017). Headache and pregnancy: A systematic review. *Journal of Headache and Pain*. https://doi.org/10.1186/s10194-017-0816-0.

36    Kumar, R., Hayhurst, K.L. and Robson, A.K. (2011). Ear, nose, and throat manifesta-
      tions during pregnancy. *Otolaryngology – Head and Neck Surgery*, 145(2), pp.188–198.

37    Hamonet, C., Delarue, M., Lefevre, J., Rottembourg, J. and Zeitoun, J. (2021).
      Ehlers-Danlos Syndrome (EDS): A common and often disregarded cause of serious
      gastrointestinal complications in children and adults. *Scholarly Journal of Otolar-
      yngology*. https://doi.org/10.32474/SJO.2021.07.000256.

38    Raines, D.A. and Cooper, D.B. (2019). Braxton Hicks contractions. In *Statpearls*.
      Treasure Island, FL: Statpearl Publishing. Accessed on 11/04/2023 at www.ncbi.nlm.
      nih.gov/books/NBK470546.

39    Karthikeyan, A. and Venkat-Raman, N. (2018). Hypermobile Ehlers–Danlos syn-
      drome and pregnancy. *Obstetric Medicine*, 11(3), pp.104–109.

40    Poole, C.J. (1986). Fatigue during the first trimester of pregnancy. *Journal of Obstetric,
      Gynecologic and Neonatal Nursing*, 15(5), pp.375–379.

41    Hakim, A., De Wandele, I., O'Callaghan, C., Pocinki, A. and Rowe, P. (2017). Chronic
      fatigue in Ehlers-Danlos syndrome – hypermobile type. *American Journal of Medical
      Genetics Part C: Seminars in Medical Genetics*, 175(1), pp.175–180.

42    Morrison, J. (2017). Managing fatigue, sleeping problems and brain fog. Ehlers-
      Danlos Support UK. Accessed on 11/04/2023 at www.ehlers-danlos.org/information/
      managing-fatigue-sleeping-problems-and-brain-fog.

43    Harris, J., Ghali, N. and van Dijk, F. (2017). Side by side – vascular EDS and hyper-
      mobile EDS compared. Ehlers-Danlos Support UK. Accessed on 11/04/2023 at www.
      ehlers-danlos.org/information/side-by-side-vascular-eds-and-hypermobile-eds-
      compared.

## CHAPTER 10

1     Pezaro, D.S., Pearce, D.G. and Reinhold, D.E. (2020). Understanding hypermobile
      Ehlers-Danlos syndrome and hypermobility spectrum disorders in the context of
      childbearing: An international qualitative study. *Midwifery*, 88, 102749.

2     Boeldt, D.S. and Bird, I.M. (2017). Vascular adaptation in pregnancy and endothelial
      dysfunction in preeclampsia. *Journal of Endocrinology*, 232(1), pp.R27–R44.

3     Pezaro, D.S., Pearce, D.G. and Reinhold, D.E. (2020). Understanding hypermobile
      Ehlers-Danlos syndrome and hypermobility spectrum disorders in the context of
      childbearing: An international qualitative study. *Midwifery*, 88, 102749. Accessed
      on 25/05/2023 at https://hedstogether.com/wp-content/uploads/2020/09/
      Post-print-EDS-maternity-interview-paper.pdf.

4     Won, C.H.J. (2015). Sleeping for two: The great paradox of sleep in pregnancy. *Journal
      of Clinical Sleep Medicine*. https://doi.org/10.5664/jcsm.4760.

5     Tinkle, B., Castori, M., Berglund, B., Cohen, H. *et al.* (2017). Hypermobile Ehlers-
      Danlos syndrome (a.k.a. Ehlers-Danlos syndrome type III and Ehlers-Danlos
      syndrome hypermobility type): Clinical description and natural history. *American
      Journal of Medical Genetics Part C: Seminars in Medical Genetics*, 175(1), pp.48–69.

6     Martín-Santos, R., Bulbena, A., Porta, M., Gago, J., Molina, L. and Duró, J.C. (1998).
      Association between joint hypermobility syndrome and panic disorder. *American
      Journal of Psychiatry*, 155(11), pp.1578–1583.

Gurer, G., Sendur, F., Gultekin, B.K. and Ozcan, M.E. (2010). The anxiety between individuals with and without joint hypermobility. *European Journal of Psychiatry*, 24(4), pp.205–209.

Murray, B., Yashar, B.M., Uhlmann, W.R., Clauw, D.J. and Petty, E.M. (2013). Ehlers-Danlos syndrome, hypermobility type: A characterization of the patients' lived experience. *American Journal of Medical Genetics Part A*, 161(12), pp.2981–2988.

7   Pezaro, S., Pearce, G. and Reinhold, E. (2018). Hypermobile Ehlers-Danlos syndrome during pregnancy, birth and beyond. *British Journal of Midwifery*, 26(4), pp.217–223.

8   Samant, H. and Kothadia, J.P. (2020). Spider angioma. In *Statpearls*. Treasure Island, FL: Statpearl Publishing. Accessed on 11/04/2023 at www.ncbi.nlm.nih.gov/books/NBK507818.

9   Burrows, N. (2016). The skin in hypermobile Ehlers-Danlos syndrome. Ehlers-Danlos Support UK. Accessed on 11/04/2023 at www.ehlers-danlos.org/information/the-skin-in-hypermobile-ehlers-danlos-syndrome.

    Castori, M. (2012). Ehlers-Danlos syndrome, hypermobility type: An underdiagnosed hereditary connective tissue disorder with mucocutaneous, articular, and systemic manifestations. *ISRN Dermatology*. https://doi.org/10.5402/2012/751768.

10  Harris, J., Ghali, N. and van Dijk, F. (2017). Side by side – vascular EDS and hypermobile EDS compared. Ehlers-Danlos Support UK. Accessed on 11/04/2023 at www.ehlers-danlos.org/information/side-by-side-vascular-eds-and-hypermobile-eds-compared.

11  Royal College of Obstetricians and Gynaecologists (RCOG) (2015). Reducing the Risk of Venous Thromboembolism during Pregnancy and the Puerperium. Green-top Guideline No. 37a. Accessed on 11/04/2023 at www.rcog.org.uk/media/qejfhcaj/gtg-37a.pdf.

12  Zamponi, V., Mazzilli, R., Mazzilli, F. and Fantini, M. (2021). Effect of sex hormones on human voice physiology: From childhood to senescence. *Hormones*. https://doi.org/10.1007/s42000-021-00298-y.

13  Hunter, A. (2017). Speech, language, voice and swallowing in the Ehlers-Danlos syndromes. Ehlers-Danlos Support UK. Accessed on 11/04/2023 at www.ehlers-danlos.org/information/speech-language-voice-and-swallowing-in-the-ehlers-danlos-syndromes.

14  National Institute for Health and Care Excellence (NICE) (2021). Recommendations. NG201. Accessed on 11/04/2023 at www.nice.org.uk/guidance/ng201/chapter/Recommendations#routine-antenatal-clinical-care.

15  Karthikeyan, A. and Venkat-Raman, N. (2018). Hypermobile Ehlers–Danlos syndrome and pregnancy. *Obstetric Medicine*, 11(3), pp.104–109.

## CHAPTER 11

1   National Institute for Health and Care Excellence (NICE) (2021). Schedule of Antenatal Appointments. NG201. Accessed on 11/04/2023 at www.nice.org.uk/guidance/ng201/resources/schedule-of-antenatal-appointments-pdf-9204300829.

2   Sundelin, H.E.K., Stephansson, O., Johansson, K. and Ludvigsson, J.F. (2016). Pregnancy outcome in joint hypermobility syndrome and Ehlers-Danlos syndrome. *Acta Obstetricia et Gynecologica Scandinavica*, 96(1), pp.114–119.

Castori, M., Morlino, S., Dordoni, C., Celletti, C. *et al.* (2012). Gynecologic and obstetric implications of the joint hypermobility syndrome (a.k.a. Ehlers-Danlos syndrome hypermobility type) in 82 Italian patients. *American Journal of Medical Genetics Part A*, 158A(9), pp.2176–2182.

3    Castori, M., Morlino, S., Dordoni, C., Celletti, C. *et al.* (2012). Gynecologic and obstetric implications of the joint hypermobility syndrome (a.k.a. Ehlers-Danlos syndrome hypermobility type) in 82 Italian patients. *American Journal of Medical Genetics Part A*, 158A(9), pp.2176–2182.

Simionescu, A.A., Cirstoiu, M.M., Cirstoiu, C., Stanescu, A.M.A. and Crețu, B. (2021). Current evidence about developmental dysplasia of the hip in pregnancy. *Medicina*, 57(7), 655.

Sastry, R., Sufianov, R., Laviv, Y., Young, B.C. *et al.* (2020). Chiari I malformation and pregnancy: A comprehensive review of the literature to address common questions and to guide management. *Acta Neurochirurgica*, 162(7), pp.1565–1573.

Furuta, N., Kondoh, E., Yamada, S., Kawasaki, K. *et al.* (2013). Vaginal delivery in the presence of huge vulvar varicosities: A case report with MRI evaluation. *European Journal of Obstetrics, Gynecology, and Reproductive Biology*, 167(2), pp.127–131.

4    Wiesmann, T., Castori, M., Malfait, F. and Wulf, H. (2014). Recommendations for anesthesia and perioperative management in patients with Ehlers-Danlos syndrome(s). *Orphanet Journal of Rare Diseases*. https://doi.org/10.1186/s13023-014-0109-5.

5    Schubart, J.R., Schaefer, E., Janicki, P., Adhikary, S.D. *et al.* (2019). Resistance to local anesthesia in people with the Ehlers-Danlos syndromes presenting for dental surgery. *Journal of Dental Anesthesia and Pain Medicine*, 19(5), pp.261–270.

Arendt-Nielsen, L., Kaalund, S., Bjerring, P. and Høgsaa, B. (1990). Insufficient effect of local analgesics in Ehlers Danlos type III patients (connective tissue disorder). *Acta Anaesthesiologica Scandinavica*, 34(5), pp.358–361.

6    De Costa, P.J., Van den Berghe, L.I. and Martens, L.C. (2005). Generalized joint hypermobility and temporomandibular disorders: Inherited connective tissue disease as a model with maximum expression. *Journal of Orofacial Pain*, 19(1), pp 47–57.

7    Moran, F. (2021). Statement on the use of opioids in pain management of the Ehlers-Danlos syndromes and hypermobility spectrum disorders. Ehlers Danlos Society. Accessed on 31/01/2023 at www.ehlers-danlos.com/statement-on-the-use-of-opioids-in-pain-management-of-the-ehlers-danlos-syndromes-and-hypermobility-spectrum-disorders.

8    Epstein, M., Song, B., Yeh, P., Nguyen, D. and Harrell, J. (n.d.). *Ehlers Danlos Syndrome: A Retrospective Review of the Current Treatment Options in Pain Management*. Accessed on 31/01/2023 at www.texaspain.org/assets/2019AnnualMeeting/EpsteinEDS_Retrospective_Review.pdf.

9    Bachmutsky, I., Wei, X.P., Kish, E. and Yackle, K. (2020). Opioids depress breathing through two small brainstem sites. *eLife*, 9, p.e52694.

10   Martín-Santos, R., Bulbena, A., Porta, M., Gago, J., Molina, L. and Duró, J.C. (1998). Association between joint hypermobility syndrome and panic disorder. *American Journal of Psychiatry*, 155(11), pp.1578–1583.

Murray, B., Yashar, B.M., Uhlmann, W.R., Clauw, D.J. and Petty, E.M. (2013). Ehlers-Danlos syndrome, hypermobility type: A characterization of the patients' lived experience. *American Journal of Medical Genetics Part A*, 161(12), pp.2981–2988.

11  Faisal-Cury, A. and Menezes, P.R. (2012). Antenatal depression strongly predicts postnatal depression in primary health care. *Revista Brasileira de Psiquiatria*, 34(4), pp.446–450.

Leigh, B. and Milgrom, J. (2008). Risk factors for antenatal depression, postnatal depression and parenting stress. *BMC Psychiatry*. https://doi.org/10.1186/1471-244x-8-24.

12  Pocinki, A. (2016). Webinar: 'Psychiatric misdiagnoses in EDS: When is anxiety not anxiety?' [Video file]. EDS Awareness. Accessed on 30/01/2023 at www.chronicpain-partners.com/webinar/free-webinar-psychiatric-misdiagnoses-eds-anxiety-not-anxiety.

13  Jiménez-Encarnación, E. and Vilá, L.M. (2013). Recurrent venous thrombosis in Ehlers-Danlos syndrome type III: An atypical manifestation. *Case Reports*. http://dx.doi.org/10.1136/bcr-2013-008922.

14  Hamonet, C., Delarue, M., Lefevre, J., Rottembourg, J. and Zeitoun, J. (2021). Ehlers-Danlos syndrome (EDS): A common and often disregarded cause of serious gastrointestinal complications in children and adults. *Scholarly Journal of Otolaryngology*. https://doi.org/10.32474/SJO.2021.07.000256.

15  Clayton, H.A., Jones, S.A.H. and Henriques, D.Y.P. (2015). Proprioceptive precision is impaired in Ehlers–Danlos syndrome. *SpringerPlus*. https://doi.org/10.1186/s40064-015-1089-1.

16  Karthikeyan, A. and Venkat-Raman, N. (2018). Hypermobile Ehlers–Danlos syndrome and pregnancy. *Obstetric Medicine*, 11(3), pp.104–109.

Ali, A., Andrzejowski, P., Kanakaris, N.K. and Giannoudis, P.V. (2020). Pelvic girdle pain, hypermobility spectrum disorder and hypermobility-type Ehlers-Danlos syndrome: A narrative literature review. *Journal of Clinical Medicine*, 9(12), 3992.

17  Karthikeyan, A. and Venkat-Raman, N. (2018). Hypermobile Ehlers–Danlos syndrome and pregnancy. *Obstetric Medicine*, 11(3), pp.104–109.

18  Ahlqvist, K., Bjelland, E.K., Pingel, R., Schlager, A., Nilsson-Wikmar, L. and Kristiansson, P. (2020). The association of self-reported generalized joint hypermobility with pelvic girdle pain during pregnancy: A retrospective cohort study. *BMC Musculoskeletal Disorders*. https://doi.org/10.1186/s12891-020-03486-w.

Royal College of Obstetricians and Gynaecologists (RCOG) (n.d.). Pelvic Girdle Pain and Pregnancy. Accessed on 11/04/2023 at www.rcog.org.uk/for-the-public/browse-all-patient-information-leaflets/pelvic-girdle-pain-and-pregnancy.

Mukkannavar, P., Desai, B.R., Mohanty, U., Parvatikar, V., Karwa, D. and Daiwajna, S. (2013). Pelvic girdle pain after childbirth: The impact of mode of delivery. *Journal of Back and Musculoskeletal Rehabilitation*, 26(3), pp.281–290.

19  Royal College of Obstetricians and Gynaecologists (RCOG) (2017). Management of breech presentation. *BJOG: International Journal of Obstetrics and Gynaecology*, 124(7), pp.e151–e177.

Goffinet, F., Carayol, M., Foidart, J.-M., Alexander, S. *et al.* (2006). Is planned vaginal delivery for breech presentation at term still an option? Results of an observational prospective survey in France and Belgium. *American Journal of Obstetrics and Gynecology*, 194(4), pp.1002–1011.

20  Lind, J. and Wallenburg, H.C.S. (2002). Pregnancy and the Ehlers-Danlos syndrome: A retrospective study in a Dutch population. *Acta Obstetricia et Gynecologica Scandinavica*, 81(4), pp.293–300.

21  Lind, J. and Wallenburg, H.C.S. (2002). Pregnancy and the Ehlers-Danlos syndrome: A retrospective study in a Dutch population. *Acta Obstetricia et Gynecologica Scandinavica*, 81(4), pp.293–300.

22  Knoepp, L.R., McDermott, K.C., Muñoz, A., Blomquist, J.L. and Handa, V.L. (2012). Joint hypermobility, obstetrical outcomes, and pelvic floor disorders. *International Urogynecology Journal*, 24(5), pp.735–740.

Tinkle, B., Castori, M., Berglund, B., Cohen, H. *et al.* (2017). Hypermobile Ehlers-Danlos syndrome (a.k.a. Ehlers-Danlos syndrome type III and Ehlers-Danlos syndrome hypermobility type): Clinical description and natural history. *American Journal of Medical Genetics Part C: Seminars in Medical Genetics*, 175(1), pp.48–69.

23  Lind, J. and Wallenburg, H.C.S. (2002). Pregnancy and the Ehlers-Danlos syndrome: A retrospective study in a Dutch population. *Acta Obstetricia et Gynecologica Scandinavica*, 81(4), pp.293–300.

Pagon, R., Bird, T. and Dolan, C. (1993). Ehlers-Danlos syndrome, hypermobility type. Accessed on 01/02/2023 at www.rareconnect.org/uploads/documents/ehlers-danlos-syndrome-hypermobility-type.pdf.

24  Hugon-Rodin, J., Lebègue, G., Becourt, S., Hamonet, C. and Gompel, A. (2016). Gynecologic symptoms and the influence on reproductive life in 386 women with hypermobility type Ehlers-Danlos syndrome: A cohort study. *Orphanet Journal of Rare Diseases*. https://doi.org/10.1186/s13023-016-0511-2.

Hamonet, C., Delarue, M., Lefevre, J., Rottembourg, J. and Zeitoun, J. (2021). Ehlers-Danlos syndrome (EDS) : A common and often disregarded cause of serious gastrointestinal complications in children and adults. *Scholarly Journal of Otolaryngology*. https://doi.org/10.32474/SJO.2021.07.000256.

25  Pagon, R., Bird, T. and Dolan, C. (1993). Ehlers-Danlos syndrome, hypermobility type. Accessed on 01/02/2023 at www.rareconnect.org/uploads/documents/ehlers-danlos-syndrome-hypermobility-type.pdf.

26  Chen, Q., Qiu, X., Fu, A. and Han, Y. (2022). Effect of prenatal perineal massage on postpartum perineal injury and postpartum complications: A meta-analysis. *Computational and Mathematical Methods in Medicine*, 2022, pp.1–10.

27  Knoepp, L.R., McDermott, K.C., Muñoz, A., Blomquist, J.L. and Handa, V.L. (2012). Joint hypermobility, obstetrical outcomes, and pelvic floor disorders. *International Urogynecology Journal*, 24(5), pp.735–740.

Tinkle, B., Castori, M., Berglund, B., Cohen, H. *et al.* (2017). Hypermobile Ehlers-Danlos syndrome (a.k.a. Ehlers-Danlos syndrome type III and Ehlers-Danlos syndrome hypermobility type): Clinical description and natural history. *American Journal of Medical Genetics Part C: Seminars in Medical Genetics*, 175(1), pp.48–69.

28  Bell, C.H., Muggleton, S. and Davis, D.L. (2022). Birth plans: A systematic, integrative review into their purpose, process, and impact. *Midwifery*, 111, 103388.

29  Brooks, K. (2017). Impacts of Birth Plans on Maternal Satisfaction a Literature Review and Focus Group Study. Senior Honors Projects, 2010–2019. Accessed on 11/04/2023 at https://commons.lib.jmu.edu/honors201019/309.

30 Divall, B., Spiby, H., Nolan, M. and Slade, P. (2017). Plans, preferences or going with the flow: An online exploration of women's views and experiences of birth plans. *Midwifery*, 54, pp.29–34.

31 Lind, J. and Wallenburg, H.C.S. (2002). Pregnancy and the Ehlers-Danlos syndrome: A retrospective study in a Dutch population. *Acta Obstetricia et Gynecologica Scandinavica*, 81(4), pp.293–300.

32 Lind, J. and Wallenburg, H.C.S. (2002). Pregnancy and the Ehlers-Danlos syndrome: A retrospective study in a Dutch population. *Acta Obstetricia et Gynecologica Scandinavica*, 81(4), pp.293–300.

33 Knoepp, L.R., McDermott, K.C., Muñoz, A., Blomquist, J.L. and Handa, V.L. (2012). Joint hypermobility, obstetrical outcomes, and pelvic floor disorders. *International Urogynecology Journal*, 24(5), pp.735–740.

34 Lind, J. and Wallenburg, H.C.S. (2002). Pregnancy and the Ehlers-Danlos syndrome: A retrospective study in a Dutch population. *Acta Obstetricia et Gynecologica Scandinavica*, 81(4), pp.293–300.

35 Castori, M., Morlino, S., Dordoni, C., Celletti, C. *et al.* (2012). Gynecologic and obstetric implications of the joint hypermobility syndrome (a.k.a. Ehlers-Danlos syndrome hypermobility type) in 82 Italian patients. *American Journal of Medical Genetics Part A*, 158A(9), pp.2176–2182.

36 Esegbona, G. (2018). Advances in birth positioning [Video file]. Maternity and Midwifery Forum. Accessed on 01/02/2023 at https://youtu.be/E5PiNozW7oo.

37 Tinkle, B., Castori, M., Berglund, B., Cohen, H. *et al.* (2017). Hypermobile Ehlers-Danlos syndrome (a.k.a. Ehlers-Danlos syndrome type III and Ehlers-Danlos syndrome hypermobility type): Clinical description and natural history. *American Journal of Medical Genetics Part C: Seminars in Medical Genetics*, 175(1), pp.48–69.

38 Tinkle, B., Castori, M., Berglund, B., Cohen, H. *et al.* (2017). Hypermobile Ehlers-Danlos syndrome (a.k.a. Ehlers-Danlos syndrome type III and Ehlers-Danlos syndrome hypermobility type): Clinical description and natural history. *American Journal of Medical Genetics Part C: Seminars in Medical Genetics*, 175(1), pp.48–69.

39 Pagon, R., Bird, T. and Dolan, C. (1993). Ehlers-Danlos syndrome, hypermobility type. Accessed on 01/02/2023 at www.rareconnect.org/uploads/documents/ehlers-danlos-syndrome-hypermobility-type.pdf.

40 Castori, M., Morlino, S., Dordoni, C., Celletti, C. *et al.* (2012). Gynecologic and obstetric implications of the joint hypermobility syndrome (a.k.a. Ehlers-Danlos syndrome hypermobility type) in 82 Italian patients. *American Journal of Medical Genetics Part A*, 158A(9), pp.2176–2182.

41 Hugon-Rodin, J., Lebègue, G., Becourt, S., Hamonet, C. and Gompel, A. (2016). Gynecologic symptoms and the influence on reproductive life in 386 women with hypermobility type Ehlers-Danlos syndrome: A cohort study. *Orphanet Journal of Rare Diseases*. https://doi.org/10.1186/s13023-016-0511-2.

42 Nove, A., Berrington, A. and Matthews, Z. (2012). Comparing the odds of postpartum haemorrhage in planned home birth against planned hospital birth: Results of an observational study of over 500,000 maternities in the UK. *BMC Pregnancy and Childbirth*. https://doi.org/10.1186/1471-2393-12-130.

43 Deneux-Tharaux, C., Sentilhes, L., Maillard, F., Closset, E. *et al.* (2013). Effect of routine controlled cord traction as part of the active management of the third stage

of labour on postpartum haemorrhage: Multicentre randomised controlled trial (TRACOR). *BMJ*. https://doi.org/10.1136/bmj.f1541.

44  Dekker, R. (2019). Evidence on: The Vitamin K Shot in Newborns. Evidence Based Birth®. Accessed on 11/04/2023 at https://evidencebasedbirth.com/evidence-for-the-vitamin-k-shot-in-newborns.

Busfield, A., McNinch, A. and Tripp, J. (2007). Neonatal vitamin K prophylaxis in Great Britain and Ireland: The impact of perceived risk and product licensing on effectiveness. *Archives of Disease in Childhood*, 92(9), pp.754–758.

Fear, N.T., Roman, E., Ansell, P., Simpson, J., Day, N. and Eden, O.B. (2003). Vitamin K and childhood cancer: A report from the United Kingdom Childhood Cancer Study. *British Journal of Cancer*, 89(7), pp.1228–1231.

45  World Health Organization (2018). *Intrapartum Care for a Positive Childbirth Experience*. Accessed on 11/04/2023 at https://apps.who.int/iris/bitstream/handle/10665/260178/9789241550215-eng.pdf.

## CHAPTER 12

1  Sundelin, H.E.K., Stephansson, O., Johansson, K. and Ludvigsson, J.F. (2016). Pregnancy outcome in joint hypermobility syndrome and Ehlers-Danlos syndrome. *Acta Obstetricia et Gynecologica Scandinavica*, 96(1), pp.114–119.

Lind, J. and Wallenburg, H.C.S. (2002). Pregnancy and the Ehlers-Danlos syndrome: A retrospective study in a Dutch population. *Acta Obstetricia et Gynecologica Scandinavica*, 81(4), pp.293–300.

Dutta, I., Wilson, H. and Oteri, O. (2011). Pregnancy and delivery in Ehlers-Danlos syndrome (hypermobility type): Review of the literature. *Obstetrics and Gynecology International*. https://doi.org/10.1155/2011/306413.

Hugon-Rodin, J., Lebègue, G., Becourt, S., Hamonet, C. and Gompel, A. (2016). Gynecologic symptoms and the influence on reproductive life in 386 women with hypermobility type Ehlers-Danlos syndrome: A cohort study. *Orphanet Journal of Rare Diseases*. https://doi.org/10.1186/s13023-016-0511-2.

2  Castori, M., Morlino, S., Dordoni, C., Celletti, C. *et al.* (2012). Gynecologic and obstetric implications of the joint hypermobility syndrome (a.k.a. Ehlers-Danlos syndrome hypermobility type) in 82 Italian patients. *American Journal of Medical Genetics Part A*, 158A(9), pp.2176–2182.

3  Muñoz-de-Toro, M., Varayoud, J., Ramos, J., Rodríguez, H. and Luque, E. (2003). Collagen remodelling during cervical ripening is a key event for successful vaginal delivery. *Brazilian Journal of Morphological Sciences*, 20(2), pp.75–84.

4  Gilliam, E., Hoffman, J.D. and Yeh, G. (2020). Urogenital and pelvic complications in the Ehlers-Danlos syndromes and associated hypermobility spectrum disorders: A scoping review. *Clinical Genetics*, 97(1), pp.168–178.

5  Gilliam, E., Hoffman, J.D. and Yeh, G. (2020). Urogenital and pelvic complications in the Ehlers-Danlos syndromes and associated hypermobility spectrum disorders: A scoping review. *Clinical Genetics*, 97(1), pp.168–178.

6  Berglund, B. and Björck, E. (2012). Women with Ehlers-Danlos syndrome experience low oral health-related quality of life. *Journal of Orofacial Pain*, 26(4), pp.307–314.

7   Lind, J. and Wallenburg, H.C.S. (2002). Pregnancy and the Ehlers-Danlos syndrome: A retrospective study in a Dutch population. *Acta Obstetricia et Gynecologica Scandinavica*, 81(4), pp.293–300.

8   Alexander, J.M. and Cox, S.M. (1996). Clinical course of premature rupture of the membranes. *Seminars in Perinatology*, 20(5), pp.369–374.

9   Patel, R.R. (2004). Does gestation vary by ethnic group? A London-based study of over 122 000 pregnancies with spontaneous onset of labour. *International Journal of Epidemiology*, 33(1), pp.107–113.

10  American College of Obstetricians and Gynecologists (2013). ACOG Committee Opinion No 579: Definition of term pregnancy. *Obstetrics and Gynecology*, 122(5), pp.1139–1140.

11  Weekes, A.R. and Flynn, M.J. (1975). Engagement of the fetal head in primigravidae and its relationship to duration of gestation and time of onset of labour. *British Journal of Obstetrics and Gynaecology*, 82(1), pp.7–11.

12  Sundelin, H.E.K., Stephansson, O., Johansson, K. and Ludvigsson, J.F. (2016). Pregnancy outcome in joint hypermobility syndrome and Ehlers-Danlos syndrome. *Acta Obstetricia et Gynecologica Scandinavica*, 96(1), pp.114–119.

Lind, J. and Wallenburg, H.C.S. (2002). Pregnancy and the Ehlers-Danlos syndrome: A retrospective study in a Dutch population. *Acta Obstetricia et Gynecologica Scandinavica*, 81(4), pp.293–300.

Hugon-Rodin, J., Lebègue, G., Becourt, S., Hamonet, C. and Gompel, A. (2016). Gynecologic symptoms and the influence on reproductive life in 386 women with hypermobility type Ehlers-Danlos syndrome: A cohort study. *Orphanet Journal of Rare Diseases*. https://doi.org/10.1186/s13023-016-0511-2.

Castori, M., Morlino, S., Dordoni, C., Celletti, C. *et al.* (2012). Gynecologic and obstetric implications of the joint hypermobility syndrome (a.k.a. Ehlers-Danlos syndrome hypermobility type) in 82 Italian patients. *American Journal of Medical Genetics Part A*, 158A(9), pp.2176–2182.

13  Tilden, E.L., Phillippi, J.C., Ahlberg, M., King, T.L. *et al.* (2019). Describing latent phase duration and associated characteristics among 1281 low-risk women in spontaneous labor. *Birth*, 46(4), pp.592–601.

14  Tilden, E.L., Phillippi, J.C., Ahlberg, M., King, T.L. *et al.* (2019). Describing latent phase duration and associated characteristics among 1281 low-risk women in spontaneous labor. *Birth*, 46(4), pp.592–601.

15  Jansen, L., Gibson, M., Bowles, B.C. and Leach, J. (2013). First do no harm: Interventions during childbirth. *Journal of Perinatal Education*, 22(2), pp.83–92.

16  Pezaro, D.S., Pearce, D.G. and Reinhold, D.E. (2020). Understanding hypermobile Ehlers-Danlos syndrome and hypermobility spectrum disorders in the context of childbearing: An international qualitative study. *Midwifery*, 88, 102749.

17  Dencker, A., Berg, M., Bergqvist, L. and Lilja, H. (2010). Identification of latent phase factors associated with active labor duration in low-risk nulliparous women with spontaneous contractions. *Acta Obstetricia et Gynecologica Scandinavica*, 89(8), pp.1034–1039.

18  Labor, S. and Maguire, S. (2008). The pain of labour. *Reviews in Pain*, 2(2), pp.15–19.

Ullman, R., Smith, L.A., Burns, E., Mori, R. and Dowswell, T. (2010). Parenteral opioids for maternal pain management in labour. *Cochrane Database of Systematic Reviews.* https://doi.org/10.1002/14651858.cd007396.pub2.

19    Lind, J. and Wallenburg, H.C.S. (2002). Pregnancy and the Ehlers-Danlos syndrome: A retrospective study in a Dutch population. *Acta Obstetricia et Gynecologica Scandinavica*, 81(4), pp.293-300.

Pagon, R., Bird, T. and Dolan, C. (1993). Ehlers-Danlos syndrome, hypermobility type. Accessed on 01/02/2023 at www.rareconnect.org/uploads/documents/ehlers-danlos-syndrome-hypermobility-type.pdf.

20    Bohren, M.A., Hofmeyr, G.J., Sakala, C., Fukuzawa, R.K. and Cuthbert, A. (2017). Continuous support for women during childbirth. *Cochrane Database of Systematic Reviews.* https://doi.org/10.1002/14651858.CD003766.pub6.

21    Yang, L., Yi, T., Zhou, M., Wang, C. *et al.* (2020). Clinical effectiveness of position management and manual rotation of the fetal position with a U-shaped birth stool for vaginal delivery of a fetus in a persistent occiput posterior position. *Journal of International Medical Research.* https://doi.org/10.1177/0300060520924275.

Kibuka, M., Price, A., Onakpoya, I., Tierney, S. and Clarke, M. (2021). Evaluating the effects of maternal positions in childbirth: An overview of Cochrane Systematic Reviews. *European Journal of Midwifery*, 5, pp.1-14.

22    Kibuka, M., Price, A., Onakpoya, I., Tierney, S. and Clarke, M. (2021). Evaluating the effects of maternal positions in childbirth: An overview of Cochrane Systematic Reviews. *European Journal of Midwifery*, 5, pp.1-14.

23    Kamala, B.A., Kidanto, H., Wangwe, P., Dalen, I. *et al.* (2018). Intrapartum fetal heart rate monitoring using a handheld Doppler versus Pinard stethoscope: A randomized controlled study in Dar es Salaam. *International Journal of Women's Health*, 10, pp.341-348.

24    Dencker, A., Berg, M., Bergqvist, L. and Lilja, H. (2010). Identification of latent phase factors associated with active labor duration in low-risk nulliparous women with spontaneous contractions. *Acta Obstetricia et Gynecologica Scandinavica*, 89(8), pp.1034-1039.

Singata, M., Tranmer, J. and Gyte, G.M. (2010). Restricting oral fluid and food intake during labour. *Cochrane Database of Systematic Reviews.* https://doi.org/10.1002/14651858.cd003930.pub2.

Ozkan, S., Kadioglu, M. and Rathfisch, G. (2017). Restricting oral fluid and food intake during labour: A qualitative analysis of women's views. *International Journal of Caring Sciences*, 10(1), pp.235-242. Accessed on 11/04/2023 at www.internationaljournalofcaringsciences.org/docs/27_aydin_original_10_1.pdf.

25    Raines, D.A. and Cooper, D.B. (2019). Braxton Hicks contractions. In *Statpearls.* Treasure Island, FL: Statpearl Publishing. Accessed on 11/04/2023 at www.ncbi.nlm.nih.gov/books/NBK470546.

26    Kerr-Wilson, R.H.J., Parham, G.P. and Orr, J.W. (1983). The effect of a full bladder on labor. *Obstetrics and Gynecology*, 62(3), pp.319-323.

27    Royal College of Obstetricians and Gynaecologists (RCOG) (2016). Prevention and management of postpartum haemorrhage. *BJOG: International Journal of Obstetrics and Gynaecology*, 124(5), pp.e106-e149.

28  Khullar, V. (2014). The bladder and EDS [Video file]. Ehlers-Danlos Support UK. Accessed on 11/04/2023 at www.ehlers-danlos.org/information/video-the-bladder-and-eds.

29  Cao, D., Rao, L., Yuan, J., Zhang, D. and Lu, B. (2022). Prevalence and risk factors of overt postpartum urinary retention among primiparous women after vaginal delivery: A case-control study. *BMC Pregnancy and Childbirth*. https://doi.org/10.1186/s12884-021-04369-1.

30  Wiesmann, T., Castori, M., Malfait, F. and Wulf, H. (2014). Recommendations for anesthesia and perioperative management in patients with Ehlers-Danlos syndrome(s). *Orphanet Journal of Rare Diseases*. https://doi.org/10.1186/s13023-014-0109-5.

31  Kaushal, R., Bhanot, A., Luthra, S., Gupta, P.N. and Sharma, R.B. (2005). Intrapartum coccygeal fracture, a cause for postpartum coccydynia: A case report. *Journal of Surgical Orthopaedic Advances*, 14(3), pp.136–137.

    Maigne, J.-Y., Rusakiewicz, F. and Diouf, M. (2012). Postpartum coccydynia: A case series study of 57 women. *European Journal of Physical and Rehabilitation Medicine*, 48(3), pp.387–392.

32  Martín-Santos, R., Bulbena, A., Porta, M., Gago, J., Molina, L. and Duró, J.C. (1998). Association between joint hypermobility syndrome and panic disorder. *American Journal of Psychiatry*, 155(11), pp.1578–1583.

    Murray, B., Yashar, B.M., Uhlmann, W.R., Clauw, D.J. and Petty, E.M. (2013). Ehlers-Danlos syndrome, hypermobility type: A characterization of the patients' lived experience. *American Journal of Medical Genetics Part A*, 161(12), pp.2981–2988.

33  World Health Organization (2018). *Intrapartum Care for a Positive Childbirth Experience*. Accessed on 11/04/2023 at https://apps.who.int/iris/bitstream/handle/10665/260178/9789241550215-eng.pdf.

    National Institute for Health and Care Excellence (NICE) (2022). Intrapartum Care for Healthy Women and Babies: 1.1 Place of Birth. CG190. Accessed on 11/04/2023 at www.nice.org.uk/guidance/cg190/chapter/Recommendations#place-of-birth.

34  National Institute for Health and Care Excellence (NICE) (2022). Intrapartum Care for Healthy Women and Babies: 1.1 Place of Birth. CG190. Accessed on 11/04/2023 at www.nice.org.uk/guidance/cg190/chapter/Recommendations#place-of-birth.

35  Hakim, A.J., Grahame, R., Norris, P. and Hopper, C. (2005). Local anaesthetic failure in joint hypermobility syndrome. *Journal of the Royal Society of Medicine*, 98(2), pp.84–85.

    Schubart, J.R., Schaefer, E., Janicki, P., Adhikary, S.D. *et al.* (2019). Resistance to local anesthesia in people with the Ehlers-Danlos syndromes presenting for dental surgery. *Journal of Dental Anesthesia and Pain Medicine*, 19(5), pp.261–270.

    Arendt-Nielsen, L., Kaalund, S., Bjerring, P. and Høgsaa, B. (1990). Insufficient effect of local analgesics in Ehlers Danlos type III patients (connective tissue disorder). *Acta Anaesthesiologica Scandinavica*, 34(5), pp.358–361.

36  Dekker, R. (2018). Breathing for pain relief during labor.Evidence Based Birth®. Accessed on 11/04/2023 at https://evidencebasedbirth.com/breathing-for-pain-relief-during-labor.

37    Royal College of Midwives (2016). Introducing sterile water injections as an alternative for pain relief [Video file]. Accessed on 01/02/2023 at www.youtube.com/watch?v=FLO2Cn8zEvs.

Mårtensson, L.B., Hutton, E.K., Lee, N., Kildea, S., Gao, Y. and Bergh, I. (2018). Sterile water injections for childbirth pain: An evidenced based guide to practice. *Women and Birth*, 31(5), pp.380–385.

Genç Koyucu, R., Demirci, N., Yumru, A.E., Salman, S. *et al.* (2018). Effects of intradermal sterile water injections in women with low back pain in labor: A randomized, controlled, clinical trial. *Balkan Medical Journal*, 35(2), pp.148–154.

38    Torkamani, S., Kangani, F. and Janani, F. (2010). The effects of delivery in water on duration of delivery and pain compared with normal delivery. *Pakistan Journal of Medical Sciences*, 26(3), pp.551–555.

Cluett, E.R. and Burns, E. (2009). Immersion in water in labour and birth. *Cochrane Database of Systematic Reviews*. https://doi.org/10.1002/14651858.cd000111.pub3.

39    Maghalian, M., Kamalifard, M., Hassanzadeh, R. and Mirghafourvand, M. (2022). The effect of massage on childbirth satisfaction: A systematic review and meta-analysis. *Advances in Integrative Medicine*. https://doi.org/10.1016/j.aimed.2022.05.002.

Field, T. (2010). Pregnancy and labor massage. *Expert Review of Obstetrics and Gynecology*, 5(2), pp.177–181.

40    Grant, E., Tao, W., Craig, M., McIntire, D. and Leveno, K. (2014). Neuraxial analgesia effects on labour progression: Facts, fallacies, uncertainties and the future. *BJOG: International Journal of Obstetrics and Gynaecology*, 122(3), pp.288–293.

41    Bertone, A.C. and Dekker, R.L. (2021). Aromatherapy in obstetrics: A critical review of the literature. *Clinical Obstetrics and Gynecology*, 64(3), pp.572–588.

42    Tabatabaeichehr, M. and Mortazavi, H. (2020). The effectiveness of aromatherapy in the management of labor pain and anxiety: A systematic review. *Ethiopian Journal of Health Sciences*. https://doi.org/10.4314/ejhs.v30i3.16.

43    Bertone, A.C. and Dekker, R.L. (2021). Aromatherapy in obstetrics: A critical review of the literature. *Clinical Obstetrics and Gynecology*, 64(3), pp.572–588.

Tabatabaeichehr, M. and Mortazavi, H. (2020). The effectiveness of aromatherapy in the management of labor pain and anxiety: A systematic review. *Ethiopian Journal of Health Sciences*. https://doi.org/10.4314/ejhs.v30i3.16.

Smith, C.A., Collins, C.T. and Crowther, C.A. (2011). Aromatherapy for pain management in labour. https://doi.org/10.1002/14651858.CD009215.

44    Johnson, K., West, T., Diana, S., Todd, J. *et al.* (2017). Use of aromatherapy to promote a therapeutic nurse environment. *Intensive and Critical Care Nursing*, 40, pp.18–25.

45    Moran, F. (2021). Statement on the use of opioids in pain management of the Ehlers-Danlos syndromes and hypermobility spectrum disorders. Ehlers Danlos Society. Accessed on 11/04/2023 at www.ehlers-danlos.com/statement-on-the-use-of-opioids-in-pain-management-of-the-ehlers-danlos-syndromes-and-hypermobility-spectrum-disorders.

Epstein, M., Song, B., Yeh, P., Nguyen, D. and Harrell, J. (n.d.). *Ehlers Danlos Syndrome: A Retrospective Review of the Current Treatment Options in Pain Management.* Accessed on 31/01/2023 at www.texaspain.org/assets/2019AnnualMeeting/EpsteinEDS_Retrospective_Review.pdf.

Bachmutsky, I., Wei, X.P., Kish, E. and Yackle, K. (2020). Opioids depress breathing through two small brainstem sites. *eLife*, 9, p.e52694.

46  Wiesmann, T., Castori, M., Malfait, F. and Wulf, H. (2014). Recommendations for anesthesia and perioperative management in patients with Ehlers-Danlos syndrome(s). *Orphanet Journal of Rare Diseases*. https://doi.org/10.1186/s13023-014-0109-5.

James, C.F. and Burnett, H. (2019). Multiple anesthetic and obstetric challenges in a laboring patient with postural orthostatic tachycardia syndrome (POTS): Acquired hemophilia and a rare seizure disorder. *Acta Anæsthesiologica Belgica,* 70(2), pp.85–89.

McEvoy, M.D., Low, P.A. and Hebbar, L. (2007). Postural orthostatic tachycardia syndrome: Anesthetic implications in the obstetric patient. *Anesthesia and Analgesia*, 104(1), pp.166–167.

47  Castori, M., Morlino, S., Dordoni, C., Celletti, C. *et al.* (2012). Gynecologic and obstetric implications of the joint hypermobility syndrome (a.k.a. Ehlers-Danlos syndrome hypermobility type) in 82 Italian patients. *American Journal of Medical Genetics Part A*, 158A(9), pp.2176–2182.

48  Hemmerich, A., Bandrowska, T. and Dumas, G.A. (2019). The effects of squatting while pregnant on pelvic dimensions: A computational simulation to understand childbirth. *Journal of Biomechanics*, 87, pp.64–74.

Desseauve, D., Fradet, L., Lacouture, P. and Pierre, F. (2019). Is there an impact of feet position on squatting birth position? An innovative biomechanical pilot study. *BMC Pregnancy and Childbirth*. https://doi.org/10.1186/s12884-019-2408-2.

49  Nasab, P.A., Loripoor, M. and Mirzale, S. (2022). Knowledge and experience of midwives and gynecologists about manual rotation of persistent occiput posterior position. Research Square. https://doi.org/10.21203/rs.3.rs-1992789/v1.

50  Phipps, H., Hyett, J.A., Kuah, S., Pardey, J. *et al.* (2021). Persistent occiput posterior position outcomes following manual rotation: A randomized controlled trial. *American Journal of Obstetrics and Gynecology MFM*, 3(2), 100306.

Reichman, O., Gdansky, E., Latinsky, B., Labi, S. and Samueloff, A. (2008). Digital rotation from occipito-posterior to occipito-anterior decreases the need for cesarean section. *European Journal of Obstetrics and Gynecology and Reproductive Biology*, 136(1), pp.25–28.

Yang, L., Yi, T., Zhou, M., Wang, C. *et al.* (2020). Clinical effectiveness of position management and manual rotation of the fetal position with a U-shaped birth stool for vaginal delivery of a fetus in a persistent occiput posterior position. *Journal of International Medical Research*. https://doi.org/10.1177/0300060520924275.

O'Brien, S., Jordan, S. and Siassakos, D. (2019). The role of manual rotation in avoiding and managing OVD. *Best Practice and Research Clinical Obstetrics and Gynaecology*, 56, pp.69–80.

51  Broberg, J.C and Caughey, A.B. (2021). A randomized controlled trial of prophylactic early manual rotation of the occiput posterior fetus at the beginning of the second stage vs expectant management. Accessed on 01/02/2023 at www.ajogmfm.org/article/S2589-9333(21)00022-7/pdf.

Elmore, C., McBroom, K. and Ellis, J. (2020). Digital and manual rotation of the persistent occiput posterior fetus. *Journal of Midwifery and Women's Health*, 65(3), pp.387–394.

52   Felker, L. (2020). Training Midwives on Rotation of the Persistent Posterior Fetus in the Second Stage of Labor Utilizing Simulation. Graduate Nursing Project. Accessed on 01/02/2023 at https://collections.lib.utah.edu/ark:/87278/s6rr7h17.

## CHAPTER 13

1   Lemos, A., Amorim, M.M., Dornelas de Andrade, A., de Souza, A.I., Cabral Filho, J.E. and Correia, J.B. (2017). Pushing/bearing down methods for the second stage of labour. *Cochrane Database of Systematic Reviews.* https://doi.org/10.1002/14651858.cd009124.pub3.

2   National Institute for Health and Care Excellence (NICE) (2022). Intrapartum Care for Healthy Women and Babies: 1.1 Place of Birth. CG190. Accessed on 11/04/2023 at www.nice.org.uk/guidance/cg190/chapter/Recommendations#place-of-birth.

3   Bosomworth, A. and Bettany-Saltikov, J.A. (2006) Just take a deep breath: A review to compare the effects of spontaneous versus directed Valsalva pushing in the second stage of labour on maternal and fetal wellbeing. *Midwifery Digest*, 16(2), pp.157–166.

4   Lemos, A., Amorim, M.M., Dornelas de Andrade, A., de Souza, A.I., Cabral Filho, J.E. and Correia, J.B. (2017). Pushing/bearing down methods for the second stage of labour. *Cochrane Database of Systematic Reviews.* https://doi.org/10.1002/14651858.cd009124.pub3.

5   Hamilton, C. (2016). Using the Valsalva technique during the second stage of labour. *British Journal of Midwifery*, 24(2), pp.90–94.

6   Schaffer, J.I., Bloom, S.L., Casey, B.M., McIntire, D.D., Nihira, M.A. and Leveno, K.J. (2005). A randomized trial of the effects of coached vs uncoached maternal pushing during the second stage of labor on postpartum pelvic floor structure and function. *American Journal of Obstetrics and Gynecology*, 192(5), pp.1692–1696.

7   Schievink, W.I., Gordon, O.K. and Tourje, J. (2004). Connective tissue disorders with spontaneous spinal cerebrospinal fluid leaks and intracranial hypotension: A prospective study. *Neurosurgery*, 54(1), pp.65–71.

Reinstein, E., Pariani, M., Bannykh, S., Rimoin, D.L. and Schievink, W.I. (2012). Connective tissue spectrum abnormalities associated with spontaneous cerebrospinal fluid leaks: A prospective study. *European Journal of Human Genetics*, 21(4), pp.386–390.

8   Goyal, V. and Srinivasan, M. (2010). Don't hold your breath. *Journal of General Internal Medicine*, 26(3), p.345.

Mokri, B. (2002). Spontaneous CSF leaks mimicking benign exertional headaches. *Cephalalgia*, 22(10), pp.780–783.

9   Khan, K. (2016). Optimal fetal positioning: A theory in tatters – time to rewrite textbooks. *BJOG: International Journal of Obstetrics and Gynaecology*, 123(13), pp.2207–2207.

Hunter, S., Hofmeyr, G.J. and Kulier, R. (2007). Hands and knees posture in late pregnancy or labour for fetal malposition (lateral or posterior). *Cochrane Database of Systematic Reviews.* https://doi.org/10.1002/14651858.cd001063.pub3.

10   Guittier, M., Othenin-Girard, V., de Gasquet, B., Irion, O. and Boulvain, M. (2016). Maternal positioning to correct occiput posterior fetal position during the first stage

of labour: A randomised controlled trial. *BJOG: International Journal of Obstetrics and Gynaecology*, 123(13), pp.2199–2207.

Wu, X., Fan, L. and Wang, Q. (2001). Correction of occipito-posterior by maternal postures during the process of labor. *Zhonghua Fu Chan Ke Za Zhi*, 36(8), pp.468–469.

11   California Maternal Quality Care Collaborative (CMQCC) (2022). Toolkit to Support Vaginal Birth and Reduce Primary Cesareans, Appendix G: Second Stage Management of Malposition. Accessed on 01/02/2023 at www.cmqcc.org/resource/3394/download.

12   Yang, L., Yi, T., Zhou, M., Wang, C. *et al.* (2020). Clinical effectiveness of position management and manual rotation of the fetal position with a U-shaped birth stool for vaginal delivery of a fetus in a persistent occiput posterior position. *Journal of International Medical Research*. https://doi.org/10.1177/0300060520924275.

13   Kerr-Wilson, R.H.J., Parham, G.P. and Orr, J.W. (1983). The effect of a full bladder on labor. *Obstetrics and Gynecology*, 62(3), pp.319–323.

Read, J.A., Miller, F.C., Yeh, S. and Platt, L.D. (1980). Urinary bladder distention: Effect on labor and uterine activity. *Obstetrics and Gynecology*, 56(5), pp.565–570.

14   Lamb, K. and Sanders, R. (2016). Bladder care in the context of motherhood: Ensuring holistic midwifery practice. *British Journal of Midwifery*, 24(6), pp.415–421.

Birch, L., Doyle, P.M., Ellis, R. and Hogard, E. (2009). Failure to void in labour: Postnatal urinary and anal incontinence. *British Journal of Midwifery*, 17(9), pp.562–566.

15   Moore, E. and Moorhead, C. (2013). Promoting normality in the management of the perineum during the second stage of labour. *British Journal of Midwifery*, 21(9), pp.616–620.

16   Aasheim, V., Nilsen, A.B.V., Reinar, L.M. and Lukasse, M. (2017). Perineal techniques during the second stage of labour for reducing perineal trauma. *Cochrane Database of Systematic Reviews*. https://doi.org/10.1002/14651858.cd006672.pub3.

17   Dahlen, H.G., Homer, C.S.E., Cooke, M., Upton, A.M., Nunn, R.A. and Brodrick, B.S. (2009). 'Soothing the ring of fire': Australian women's and midwives' experiences of using perineal warm packs in the second stage of labour. *Midwifery*, 25(2), pp.e39–e48.

18   Singata, M., Tranmer, J. and Gyte, G.M. (2010). Restricting oral fluid and food intake during labour. *Cochrane Database of Systematic Reviews*. https://doi.org/10.1002/14651858.cd003930.pub2.

19   Esegbona, G. (2021). The impact of external hip rotation during pushing on pelvic floor dysfunction and injury. ICS 2021. Accessed on 01/02/2023 at www.ics.org/2021/abstract/104.

Esegbona, G. (2021). The impact of external hip rotation during pushing on pelvic floor dysfunction and injury [Video file]. icstelevision. Accessed on 01/02/2023 at https://m.youtube.com/watch?v=cwvbQc6RNHE.

Esegbona, G. (2018). Advances in birth positioning [Video file]. Maternity and Midwifery Forum. Accessed on 01/02/2023 at https://youtu.be/E5PiN0zW700.

## CHAPTER 14

1   Lawrence Beech, B. (2004). History of episiotomy in the United Kingdom. Association for Improvement in Maternity Services, Occasional Paper. Accessed on 11/04/2023 at www.aims.org.uk/assets/media/9/history-episiotomy-in-the-uk.pdf.

2   McCandlish, R., Bowler, U., Asten, H., Berridge, G. *et al.* (1998). A randomised controlled trial of care of the perineum during second stage of normal labour. *BJOG: International Journal of Obstetrics and Gynaecology*, 105(12), pp.1262–1272.

Petrocnik, P. and Marshall, J.E. (2015). Hands-poised technique: The future technique for perineal management of second stage of labour? A modified systematic literature review. *Midwifery*, 31(2), pp.274–279.

Albers, L.L., Sedler, K.D., Bedrick, E.J., Teaf, D. and Peralta, P. (2005). Midwifery care measures in the second stage of labor and reduction of genital tract trauma at birth: A randomized trial. *Journal of Midwifery and Women's Health*, 50(5), pp.365–372.

Aquino, C.I., Saccone, G., Troisi, J., Guida, M., Zullo, F. and Berghella, V. (2020). Is Ritgen's maneuver associated with decreased perineal lacerations and pain at delivery? *Journal of Maternal-Fetal and Neonatal Medicine*, 33(18), pp.3185–3192.

3   Košec, V. (2019). Increased oasis incidence – indicator of the quality of obstetric care? *Acta Clinica Croatica*. https://doi.org/10.20471/acc.2019.58.02.22.

Ekéus, C., Nilsson, E. and Gottvall, K. (2008). Increasing incidence of anal sphincter tears among primiparas in Sweden: A population-based register study. *Acta Obstetricia et Gynecologica Scandinavica*, 87(5), pp.564–573.

4   Tinkle, B., Castori, M., Berglund, B., Cohen, H. *et al.* (2017). Hypermobile Ehlers-Danlos syndrome (a.k.a. Ehlers-Danlos syndrome type III and Ehlers-Danlos syndrome hypermobility type): Clinical description and natural history. *American Journal of Medical Genetics Part C: Seminars in Medical Genetics*, 175(1), pp.48–69.

5   Huang, J., Zang, Y., Ren, L.-H., Li, F.-J. and Lu, H. (2019). A review and comparison of common maternal positions during the second-stage of labor. *International Journal of Nursing Sciences*, 6(4), pp.460–467.

6   Huang, J., Zang, Y., Ren, L.-H., Li, F.-J. and Lu, H. (2019). A review and comparison of common maternal positions during the second-stage of labor. *International Journal of Nursing Sciences*, 6(4), pp.460–467.

7   Aquino, C.I., Guida, M., Saccone, G., Cruz, Y. *et al.* (2018). Perineal massage during labor: A systematic review and meta-analysis of randomized controlled trials. *Journal of Maternal-Fetal and Neonatal Medicine*, 33(6), pp.1051–1063.

8   Shahoei, R., Zaheri, F., Hashemi Nasab, L. and Ranaei, F. (2017). The effect of perineal massage during the second stage of birth on nulliparous women perineal: A randomization clinical trial. *Electronic Physician*, 9(10), pp.5588–5595.

9   Geranmayeh, M., Rezaei Habibabadi, Z., Fallahkish, B., Farahani, M.A., Khakbazan, Z. and Mehran, A. (2011). Reducing perineal trauma through perineal massage with Vaseline in second stage of labor. *Archives of Gynecology and Obstetrics*, 285(1), pp.77–81.

10  Geranmayeh, M., Rezaei Habibabadi, Z., Fallahkish, B., Farahani, M.A., Khakbazan, Z. and Mehran, A. (2011). Reducing perineal trauma through perineal massage with Vaseline in second stage of labor. *Archives of Gynecology and Obstetrics*, 285(1), pp.77–81.

11    Menichini, D., Mazzaro, N., Minniti, S., Ricchi, A. *et al.* (2021). Fetal head malposition and epidural analgesia in labor: A case-control study. *Journal of Maternal-Fetal and Neonatal Medicine.* https://doi.org/10.1080/14767058.2021.1890018.

12    Young, J. (1913). The cause of internal rotation of the fœtal head. *Proceedings of the Royal Society of Medicine*, 6(Obstet_Gynaecol Sect), pp.144–166.

      Nursing Awareness (2023). Mechanism of Normal Labor. Accessed on 01/02/2023 at www.nursingawareness.com/message.php?id=94.

      Dutta, A. (2021). Presentation and Mechanism of Labour. Alliance for Global Women's Medicine. Accessed on 01/02/2023 at www.glowm.com/article/heading/vol-11--labor-and-delivery--presentation-and-mechanism-of-labor/id/414323#.Y5HdPBCny-o.

13    Elmore, C., McBroom, K. and Ellis, J. (2020). Digital and manual rotation of the persistent occiput posterior fetus. *Journal of Midwifery and Women's Health*, 65(3), pp.387–394.

      Felker, L. (2020). Training Midwives on Rotation of the Persistent Posterior Fetus in the Second Stage of Labor Utilizing Simulation. Graduate Nursing Project. Accessed on 11/02/2023 at https://collections.lib.utah.edu/ark:/87278/s6rr7h17.

14    McCandlish, R., Bowler, U., Asten, H., Berridge, G. *et al.* (1998). A randomised controlled trial of care of the perineum during second stage of normal labour. *BJOG: International Journal of Obstetrics and Gynaecology*, 105(12), pp.1262–1272.

15    Rasmussen, O., Yding, A., Lauszus, F., Andersen, C., Anhøj, J. and Boris, J. (2018). Importance of individual elements for perineal protection in childbirth: An interventional, prospective trial. *American Journal of Perinatology Reports*, 8(4), pp.e289–e294.

      Laine, K., Pirhonen, T., Rolland, R. and Pirhonen, J. (2008). Decreasing the incidence of anal sphincter tears during delivery. *Obstetrics and Gynecology*, 111(5), pp.1053–1057.

      Hals, E., Øian, P., Pirhonen, T., Gissler, M. *et al.* (2010). A multicenter interventional program to reduce the incidence of anal sphincter tears. *Obstetrics and Gynecology*, 116(4), pp.901–908.

      Laine, K., Skjeldestad, F.E., Sandvik, L. and Staff, A.C. (2012). Incidence of obstetric anal sphincter injuries after training to protect the perineum: Cohort study. *BMJ Open*, 2(5), e001649.

16    Jansova, M., Kalis, V., Lobovsky, L., Hyncik, L., Karbanova, J. and Rusavy, Z. (2014). The role of thumb and index finger placement in manual perineal protection. *International Urogynecology Journal*, 25(11), pp.1533–1540.

      Kleprlikova, H., Kalis, V., Lucovnik, M., Rusavy, Z. *et al.* (2020). Manual perineal protection: The know-how and the know-why. *Acta Obstetricia et Gynecologica Scandinavica*, 99(4), pp.445–450.

17    Castori, M., Morlino, S., Dordoni, C., Celletti, C. *et al.* (2012). Gynecologic and obstetric implications of the joint hypermobility syndrome (a.k.a. Ehlers-Danlos syndrome hypermobility type) in 82 Italian patients. *American Journal of Medical Genetics Part A*, 158A(9), pp.2176–2182.

18    Esegbona, G. (2021). The impact of external hip rotation during pushing on pelvic floor dysfunction and injury. ICS 2021. Accessed on 01/02/2023 at www.ics.org/2021/abstract/104.

Esegbona, G. (2021). The impact of external hip rotation during pushing on pelvic floor dysfunction and injury [Video file]. icstelevision. Accessed on 01/02/2023 at https://m.youtube.com/watch?v=cwvbQc6RNHE.

Esegbona, G. (2018). Advances in birth positioning [Video file]. Maternity and Midwifery Forum. Accessed on 01/02/2023 at https://youtu.be/E5PiNozW7oo.

19 Stedenfeldt, M., Pirhonen, J., Blix, E., Wilsgaard, T., Vonen, B. and Øian, P. (2012). Episiotomy characteristics and risks for obstetric anal sphincter injuries: A case-control study. *BJOG: International Journal of Obstetrics and Gynaecology*, 119(6), pp.724–730.

Buckingham, M., Wong, K.W. and Andrews, V. (2022). Mediolateral episiotomies: More astute decisions and fewer acute incisions. *British Journal of Midwifery*, 30(9), pp.512–516.

20 Schubart, J.R., Schaefer, E., Janicki, P., Adhikary, S.D. *et al.* (2019). Resistance to local anesthesia in people with the Ehlers-Danlos syndromes presenting for dental surgery. *Journal of Dental Anesthesia and Pain Medicine*, 19(5), pp.261–270.

Arendt-Nielsen, L., Kaalund, S., Bjerring, P. and Høgsaa, B. (1990). Insufficient effect of local analgesics in Ehlers Danlos type III patients (connective tissue disorder). *Acta Anaesthesiologica Scandinavica*, 34(5), pp.358–361.

21 Royal College of Obstetricians and Gynaecologists (RCOG) (2015). The Management of Third- and Fourth-Degree Perineal Tears. Green-top Guideline No. 29. Accessed on 11/04/2023 at www.rcog.org.uk/media/5jeb5hzu/gtg-29.pdf.

22 Geeky Medics (2018). Mechanism of labour & fetal positions. OSCE Guide [Video file]. Accessed on 11/04/2023 at https://youtu.be/ru1a1bC4tsw.

23 Kotaska, A. and Campbell, K. (2014). Two-step delivery may avoid shoulder dystocia: Head-to-body delivery interval is less important than we think. *Journal of Obstetrics and Gynaecology Canada*, 36(8), pp.716–720.

24 Fraser, D. and Cooper, M.A. (eds) (2003). *Myles Textbook for Midwives*. Edinburgh: Churchill Livingstone.

25 Association of Radical Midwives (2002). Birth of the Shoulders. Accessed on 11/04/2023 at www.midwifery.org.uk/articles/shoulders-birth-of.

26 Aabakke, A.J.M., Willer, H. and Krebs, L. (2016). The effect of maneuvers for shoulder delivery on perineal trauma: A randomized controlled trial. *Acta Obstetricia et Gynecologica Scandinavica*, 95(9), pp.1070–1077.

27 Menticoglou, S. (2018). Shoulder dystocia: Incidence, mechanisms, and management strategies. *International Journal of Women's Health*, 10, pp.723–732.

28 Royal College of Obstetricians and Gynaecologists (RCOG) (2012). Shoulder Dystocia. Green-top Guideline No. 42, 2nd edn. Accessed on 11/04/2023 at www.rcog.org.uk/media/ewgpnmio/gtg_42.pdf.

29 Lind, J. and Wallenburg, H.C.S. (2002). Pregnancy and the Ehlers-Danlos syndrome: A retrospective study in a Dutch population. *Acta Obstetricia et Gynecologica Scandinavica*, 81(4), pp.293–300.

## CHAPTER 15

1 Castori, M., Morlino, S., Dordoni, C., Celletti, C. *et al.* (2012). Gynecologic and obstetric implications of the joint hypermobility syndrome (a.k.a. Ehlers-Danlos

syndrome hypermobility type) in 82 Italian patients. *American Journal of Medical Genetics Part A*, 158A(9), pp.2176–2182.

Lind, J. and Wallenburg, H.C.S. (2002). Pregnancy and the Ehlers-Danlos syndrome: A retrospective study in a Dutch population. *Acta Obstetricia et Gynecologica Scandinavica*, 81(4), pp.293–300.

Hugon-Rodin, J., Lebègue, G., Becourt, S., Hamonet, C. and Gompel, A. (2016). Gynecologic symptoms and the influence on reproductive life in 386 women with hypermobility type Ehlers-Danlos syndrome: A cohort study. *Orphanet Journal of Rare Diseases*. https://doi.org/10.1186/s13023-016-0511-2.

2   Reed, R., Gabriel, L. and Kearney, L. (2019). Birthing the placenta: Women's decisions and experiences. *BMC Pregnancy and Childbirth*. https://doi.org/10.1186/s12884-019-2288-5.

3   Prendiville, W.J., Harding, J.E., Elbourne, D.R. and Stirrat, G.M. (1988). The Bristol third stage trial: Active versus physiological management of third stage of labour. *BMJ*, 297(6659), pp.1295–1300.

4   Rogers, J., Wood, J., McCandlish, R., Ayers, S., Truesdale, A. and Elbourne, D. (1998). Active versus expectant management of third stage of labour: The Hinchingbrooke randomised controlled trial. *The Lancet*, 351(9104), pp.693–699.

Fahy, K., Hastie, C., Bisits, A., Marsh, C., Smith, L. and Saxton, A. (2015). Holistic physiological care compared with active management of the third stage of labour for women at low risk of postpartum haemorrhage: A cohort study. *Women and Birth*, 23(4), pp.146–152.

Davis, D., Baddock, S., Pairman, S., Hunter, M. *et al.* (2012). Risk of severe postpartum hemorrhage in low-risk childbearing women in New Zealand: Exploring the effect of place of birth and comparing third stage management of labor. *Birth*, 39(2), pp.98–105.

5   National Institute for Health and Care Excellence (NICE) (2014). Intrapartum Care for Healthy Women and Babies: 1.4 Third Stage of Labour. CG190. Accessed on 11/04/2023 at www.nice.org.uk/guidance/cg190/chapter/Recommendations#third-stage-of-labour.

World Health Organization (2018). *Intrapartum Care for a Positive Childbirth Experience*. Accessed on 11/04/2023 at https://apps.who.int/iris/bitstream/handle/10665/260178/9789241550215-eng.pdf.

6   Deneux-Tharaux, C., Sentilhes, L., Maillard, F., Closset, E. *et al.* (2013). Effect of routine controlled cord traction as part of the active management of the third stage of labour on postpartum haemorrhage: Multicentre randomised controlled trial (TRACOR). *BMJ*. https://doi.org/10.1136/bmj.f1541.

7   Nove, A., Berrington, A. and Matthews, Z. (2012). Comparing the odds of postpartum haemorrhage in planned home birth against planned hospital birth: Results of an observational study of over 500,000 maternities in the UK. *BMC Pregnancy and Childbirth*. https://doi.org/10.1186/1471-2393-12-130.

8   Mansfield, J. (2018). Improving practice and reducing significant postpartum haemorrhage through audit. *British Journal of Midwifery*, 26(1), pp.35–43.

9   Hytten, F. (1985). Blood volume changes in normal pregnancy. *Clinics in Haematology*, 14(3), pp.601–612.

10   Baker, K. and Stephenson, J. (2022). Third stage of labour management approaches and postpartum haemorrhage in midwife-led units. *British Journal of Midwifery*, 30(5), pp.250–256.

11   Royal College of Obstetricians and Gynaecologists (RCOG) (2016). Prevention and management of postpartum haemorrhage. *BJOG: International Journal of Obstetrics and Gynaecology*, 124(5), pp.e106–e149.

12   Rath, W.H. (2011). Postpartum hemorrhage – update on problems of definitions and diagnosis. *Acta Obstetricia et Gynecologica Scandinavica*, 90(5), pp.421–428.

13   Diaz, V., Abalos, E. and Carroli, G. (2018). Methods for blood loss estimation after vaginal birth. *Cochrane Database of Systematic Reviews*. https://doi.org/10.1002/14651858.cd010980.pub2.

## CHAPTER 16

1    Frohlich, J. and Kettle, C. (2015). Perineal care. *BMJ Clinical Evidence*, 2015, 1401.

2    National Institute for Health and Care Excellence (NICE) (2022). Intrapartum Care for Healthy Women and Babies. CG190. Accessed on 11/04/2023 at www.nice.org.uk/guidance/cg190/chapter/Recommendations.

     Royal College of Obstetricians and Gynaecologists (RCOG) (2004). Methods and Materials Used in Perineal Repair. Guideline No. 23. Accessed on 12/04/2023 at http://unmfm.pbworks.com/w/file/fetch/81069629/perineal_repair-RCOG.pdf.

3    Department of Health, State of Western Australia (2017). *Statewide Clinical Guidelines for Women Requesting Immersion in Water for Pain Management during Labour and/or Birth*. Perth: Health Networks Branch, Department of Health, Western Australia. Accessed on 12/04/2023 at https://ww2.health.wa.gov.au/~/media/Files/Corporate/Policy-Frameworks/Clinical-Services-Planning-and-Programs/Policy/Women-requesting-immersion-in-water-for-pain-management/Supporting/Statewide-clinical-guidelines-for-women-requesting-immersion-in-water.pdf.

     Ardizzone, S., Sparkes, J., Craske, L. and Miller, T. (2020). *Guideline for the Management of Women Requesting Immersion in Water for Active Labour and/or Birth*. Norfolk and Norwich University Hospitals NHS Trust. Accessed on 12/04/2023 at www.nnuh.nhs.uk/publication/download/water-birth-management-version-6.

     Meehan, F., Boardman, S. and Deans, M. (2020). *Use of the Pool During Labour and Birth*. Frimley Health NHS Foundation Trust. Accessed on 04/02/2023 at www.frimleyhealthandcare.org.uk/media/2318/pool-birth-guideline.pdf.

4    Department of Health, State of Western Australia (2017). *Statewide Clinical Guidelines for Women Requesting Immersion in Water for Pain Management during Labour and/or Birth*. Perth: Health Networks Branch, Department of Health, Western Australia. Accessed on 12/04/2023 at https://ww2.health.wa.gov.au/~/media/Files/Corporate/Policy-Frameworks/Clinical-Services-Planning-and-Programs/Policy/Women-requesting-immersion-in-water-for-pain-management/Supporting/Statewide-clinical-guidelines-for-women-requesting-immersion-in-water.pdf.

5    Papoutsis, D. (2020). Novel insights on the possible effects of water exposure on the structural integrity of the perineum during a waterbirth. *European Journal of Midwifery*. https://doi.org/10.18332/ejm/127263.

6   National Institute for Health and Care Excellence (NICE) (2022). Intrapartum Care for Healthy Women and Babies. CG190. Accessed on 11/04/2023 at www.nice.org. uk/guidance/cg190/chapter/Recommendations.

Royal College of Obstetricians and Gynaecologists (RCOG) (2004). Methods and Materials Used in Perineal Repair. Guideline No. 23. Accessed on 12/04/2023 at http://unmfm.pbworks.com/w/file/fetch/81069629/perineal_repair-RCOG.pdf.

7   Boyd, M.B. (2018). Non-absorbable sutures, explained. Accessed on 04/02/2023 at https://boydbiomedical.com/articles/non-absorbable-sutures-explained.

8   Tinkle, B., Castori, M., Berglund, B., Cohen, H. *et al.* (2017). Hypermobile Ehlers-Danlos syndrome (a.k.a. Ehlers-Danlos syndrome type III and Ehlers-Danlos syndrome hypermobility type): Clinical description and natural history. *American Journal of Medical Genetics Part C: Seminars in Medical Genetics*, 175(1), pp.48–69.

9   Castori, M., Morlino, S., Dordoni, C., Celletti, C. *et al.* (2012). Gynecologic and obstetric implications of the joint hypermobility syndrome (a.k.a. Ehlers-Danlos syndrome hypermobility type) in 82 Italian patients. *American Journal of Medical Genetics Part A*, 158A(9), pp.2176–2182.

10  Hajjaj, J.P. (2017). Clinical practice: Perineal suturing. *British Journal of Midwifery*, 25(5), pp.297–300.

11  Cho, S.T. and Kim, K.H. (2021). Pelvic floor muscle exercise and training for coping with urinary incontinence. *Journal of Exercise Rehabilitation*, 17(6), pp.379–387.

12  Gutiérrez, V.B., Fader, M., Monga, A. and Kitson-Reynolds, E. (2019). Lack of care? Women's experiences of maternity bladder management. *British Journal of Midwifery*, 27(1), pp.15–25.

13  Merone, L., Tsey, K., Russell, D. and Nagle, C. (2022). Sex inequalities in medical research: A systematic scoping review of the literature. *Women's Health Reports*, 3(1), pp.49–59.

Jackson, G. (2019). The female problem: How male bias in medical trials ruined women's health. *The Guardian*, 13 November. Accessed on 04/02/2023 at www.theguardian.com/lifeandstyle/2019/nov/13/the-female-problem-male-bias-in-medical-trials.

14  Royal College of Nursing (2021). *Bladder and Bowel Care in Childbirth: RCN Guidance.* Accessed on 12/04/2023 at www.rcn.org.uk/-/media/Royal-College-Of-Nursing/ Documents/Publications/2021/April/009-553.pdf.

Chauhan, G. and Tadi, P. (2020). Physiology, postpartum changes. In *Statpearls*. Treasure Island, FL: Statpearl Publishing. Accessed on 12/04/2023 at www.ncbi.nlm. nih.gov/books/NBK555904

15  National Institute for Health and Care Excellence (NICE) (2021). Postnatal Care: 1.2 Postnatal Care of the Woman. NG194. Accessed on 12/01/2023 at www.nice.org.uk/ guidance/ng194/chapter/Recommendations#postnatal-care-of-the-woman.

16  Lamb, K. and Sanders, R. (2016). Bladder care in the context of motherhood: Ensuring holistic midwifery practice. *British Journal of Midwifery*, 24(6), pp.415–421.

17  Walsh, D. (2007). Medicalization of bladder care. *British Journal of Midwifery*. https:// doi.org/10.12968/bjom.2007.15.2.22787.

18  Obs Gynae & Midwifery News (2011). Post-partum bladder care: Background, practice and complications. Accessed on 12/04/2023 at www.ogpnews.com/2011/12/ post-partum-bladder-care-background-practice-and-complications/444.

19  Hain, T.C. (2022). Ehlers-Danlos syndrome (EHD, or EDS) hypermotility type and dizziness. Accessed on 06/02/2023 at https://dizziness-and-balance.com/disorders/medical/EHD.html.

20  Howraa, A., Patrick, A.B. and Wang, L.-X. (2012). Diagnosis and management of postural orthostatic tachycardia syndrome: A brief review. *Journal of Geriatric Cardiology*, 9(1), pp.61–67.

21  Levy, A., Nnam, M., Gudesblatt, M. and Riley, B. (2020). An investigation of headaches in hypermobile Ehlers-Danlos syndrome. *Annals of Psychiatry and Clinical Neuroscience*, 3(3), 1034.

22  Schievink, W.I., Gordon, O.K. and Tourje, J. (2004). Connective tissue disorders with spontaneous spinal cerebrospinal fluid leaks and intracranial hypotension: A prospective study. *Neurosurgery*, 54(1), pp.65–71.

    Reinstein, E., Pariani, M., Bannykh, S., Rimoin, D.L. and Schievink, W.I. (2012). Connective tissue spectrum abnormalities associated with spontaneous cerebrospinal fluid leaks: A prospective study. *European Journal of Human Genetics*, 21(4), pp.386–390.

23  Goyal, V. and Srinivasan, M. (2010). Don't hold your breath. *Journal of General Internal Medicine*, 26(3), p.345.

    Mokri, B. (2002). Spontaneous CSF leaks mimicking benign exertional headaches. *Cephalalgia*, 22(10), pp.780–783.

24  Moya, E., Phiri, N., Choko, A.T., Mwangi, M.N. and Phiri, K.S. (2022). Effect of postpartum anaemia on maternal health-related quality of life: A systematic review and meta-analysis. *BMC Public Health*. https://doi.org/10.1186/s12889-022-12710-2.

25  Hugon-Rodin, J., Lebègue, G., Becourt, S., Hamonet, C. and Gompel, A. (2016). Gynecologic symptoms and the influence on reproductive life in 386 women with hypermobility type Ehlers-Danlos syndrome: A cohort study. *Orphanet Journal of Rare Diseases*. https://doi.org/10.1186/s13023-016-0511-2.

26  Soppi, E.T. (2018). Iron deficiency without anemia – a clinical challenge. *Clinical Case Reports*, 6(6), pp.1082–1086.

27  Achebe, M.M. and Gafter-Gvili, A. (2016). How I treat anemia in pregnancy: Iron, cobalamin, and folate. *Blood*, 129(8), pp.940–949.

    Pavord, S., Myers, B., Robinson, S., Allard, S., Strong, J. and Oppenheimer, C. (2012). UK guidelines on the management of iron deficiency in pregnancy. *British Journal of Haematology*, 156(5), pp.588–600.

28  Hugon-Rodin, J., Lebègue, G., Becourt, S., Hamonet, C. and Gompel, A. (2016). Gynecologic symptoms and the influence on reproductive life in 386 women with hypermobility type Ehlers-Danlos syndrome: A cohort study. *Orphanet Journal of Rare Diseases*. https://doi.org/10.1186/s13023-016-0511-2.

29  Hugon-Rodin, J., Lebègue, G., Becourt, S., Hamonet, C. and Gompel, A. (2016). Gynecologic symptoms and the influence on reproductive life in 386 women with hypermobility type Ehlers-Danlos syndrome: A cohort study. *Orphanet Journal of Rare Diseases*. https://doi.org/10.1186/s13023-016-0511-2.

30  Suresh, V., Alagesan, J. and Indrani, D. (2022). Coccydynia and disability on postpartum vaginal delivery women. Accessed on 06/02/2023 at http://eprints.intimal.edu.my/1593/1/Vol.2022_07.pdf.

Howard, P.D., Dolan, A.N., Falco, A.N., Holland, B.M., Wilkinson, C.F. and Zink, A.M. (2013). A comparison of conservative interventions and their effectiveness for coccydynia: A systematic review. *Journal of Manual and Manipulative Therapy*, 21(4), pp.213–219.

Seidman, A.J. and Siccardi, M.A. (2020). Postpartum pubic symphysis diastasis. In *Statpearls*. Treasure Island, FL: Statpearl Publishing. Accessed on 12/04/2023 at www.ncbi.nlm.nih.gov/books/NBK537043

Pauker, S.P. and Stoler, J.M. (2022). Overview of the management of Ehlers-Danlos syndromes. Accessed on 06/02/2023 at www.medilib.ir/uptodate/show/89916.

31   The Lancet (2016). Breastfeeding: Achieving the new normal. *The Lancet*. https://doi.org/10.1016/S0140-6736(16)00210-5.

32   Thompson, R., Kruske, S., Barclay, L., Linden, K., Gao, Y. and Kildea, S. (2016). Potential predictors of nipple trauma from an in-home breastfeeding programme: A cross-sectional study. *Women and Birth*, 29(4), pp.336–344.

Fitz-Desorgher, R. (2017). *Your Baby Skin to Skin*. Bath: White Ladder.

33   McKenna, J.J. and McDade, T. (2005). Why babies should never sleep alone: A review of the co-sleeping controversy in relation to SIDS, bedsharing and breast feeding. *Paediatric Respiratory Reviews*, 6(2), pp.134–152.

Fleming, P.J. and Blair, P.S. (2015). Making informed choices on co-sleeping with your baby. *BMJ*. https://doi.org/10.1136/bmj.h563

34   UNICEF (2019). *Co-sleeping and SIDS*. Accessed on 12/04/2023 at www.unicef.org.uk/babyfriendly/wp-content/uploads/sites/2/2016/07/Co-sleeping-and-SIDS-A-Guide-for-Health-Professionals.pdf.

35   Basis: Baby Sleep Info Source (n.d.). Bed-Sharing and Breastfeeding. Accessed on 06/02/2023 at www.basisonline.org.uk/hcp-bed-sharing-and-breastfeeding.

UNICEF (2016). *Bed Sharing, Infant Sleep and SIDS: Research on Infant Health*. The Baby Friendly Initiative. Accessed on 12/04/2023 at www.unicef.org.uk/babyfriendly/news-and-research/baby-friendly-research/infant-health-research/infant-health-research-bed-sharing-infant-sleep-and-sids.

36   Breastfeeding and Medication (n.d.). Home [Facebook page]. Accessed on 06/02/2023 at www.facebook.com/breastfeedingandmedication.

Hale, T.W. (2021). *Hale's Medications & Mothers' Milk 2021: A Manual of Lactational Pharmacology*. New York: Springer Publishing Company.

The Breastfeeding Network (2022). Drugs Factsheets. Accessed on 12/04/2023 at www.breastfeedingnetwork.org.uk/drugs-factsheets.

37   Castori, M. (2012). Ehlers-Danlos syndrome, hypermobility type: An underdiagnosed hereditary connective tissue disorder with mucocutaneous, articular, and systemic manifestations. *ISRN Dermatology*. https://doi.org/10.5402/2012/751768.

38   Lind, J. and Wallenburg, H.C.S. (2002). Pregnancy and the Ehlers-Danlos syndrome: A retrospective study in a Dutch population. *Acta Obstetricia et Gynecologica Scandinavica*, 81(4), pp.293–300.

Murray, K.J. and Woo, P. (2001). Benign joint hypermobility in childhood. *Rheumatology*, 40(5), pp.489–491.

Conti, R., Zanchi, C. and Barbi, E. (2021). A floppy infant without lingual frenulum and kyphoscoliosis: Ehlers Danlos syndrome case report. *Italian Journal of Pediatrics*, 47. https://doi.org/10.1186/s13052-021-00984-y.

39 Adib, N., Davies, K., Grahame, R., Woo, P. and Murray, K.J. (2005). Joint hypermobility syndrome in childhood. A not so benign multisystem disorder? *Rheumatology*, 44(6), pp.744–750.

40 Adib, N., Davies, K., Grahame, R., Woo, P. and Murray, K.J. (2005). Joint hypermobility syndrome in childhood. A not so benign multisystem disorder? *Rheumatology*, 44(6), pp.744–750.

41 Lawrence, E.J. (2005). The clinical presentation of Ehlers-Danlos syndrome. *Advances in Neonatal Care*, 5(6), pp.301–314.

42 Adib, N., Davies, K., Grahame, R., Woo, P. and Murray, K.J. (2005). Joint hypermobility syndrome in childhood. A not so benign multisystem disorder? *Rheumatology*, 44(6), pp.744–750.

43 Paige, S.L., Lechich, K.M., Tierney, E.S.S. and Collins, R.T. (2020). Cardiac involvement in classical or hypermobile Ehlers–Danlos syndrome is uncommon. *Genetics in Medicine*, 22(10), pp.1583–1588.

44 Tinkle, B., Castori, M., Berglund, B., Cohen, H. *et al.* (2017). Hypermobile Ehlers-Danlos syndrome (a.k.a. Ehlers-Danlos syndrome type III and Ehlers-Danlos syndrome hypermobility type): Clinical description and natural history. *American Journal of Medical Genetics Part C: Seminars in Medical Genetics*, 175(1), pp.48–69.

45 Wallis, W. (2014). Cardiac features of hypermobile EDS [Video file]. Ehlers-Danlos Support UK. Accessed on 05/04/2023 at www.ehlers-danlos.org/information/video-cardiac-features-of-hypermobile-eds.

Tofts, L.J., Elliott, E.J., Munns, C., Pacey, V. and Sillence, D.O. (2009). The differential diagnosis of children with joint hypermobility: A review of the literature. *Pediatric Rheumatology*, 7. https://doi.org/10.1186/1546-0096-7-1.

## CHAPTER 17

1 Bowers, J. and Cheyne, H. (2015). Reducing the length of postnatal hospital stay: Implications for cost and quality of care. *BMC Health Services Research*. https://doi.org/10.1186/s12913-015-1214-4.

2 Bowers, J. and Cheyne, H. (2015). Reducing the length of postnatal hospital stay: Implications for cost and quality of care. *BMC Health Services Research*. https://doi.org/10.1186/s12913-015-1214-4.

Yonemoto, N., Nagai, S. and Mori, R. (2021). Schedules for home visits in the early postpartum period. *Cochrane Database of Systematic Reviews*. https://doi.org/10.1002/14651858.cd009326.pub4.

3 Henderson, J. and Redshaw, M. (2017). Change over time in women's views and experiences of maternity care in England, 1995–2014: A comparison using survey data. *Midwifery*, 44, pp.35–40.

4 Bowers, J. and Cheyne, H. (2015). Reducing the length of postnatal hospital stay: Implications for cost and quality of care. *BMC Health Services Research*. https://doi.org/10.1186/s12913-015-1214-4.

Yonemoto, N., Nagai, S. and Mori, R. (2021). Schedules for home visits in the early postpartum period. *Cochrane Database of Systematic Reviews*. https://doi.org/10.1002/14651858.cd009326.pub4.

5  Bowers, J. and Cheyne, H. (2015). Reducing the length of postnatal hospital stay: Implications for cost and quality of care. *BMC Health Services Research*. https://doi.org/10.1186/s12913-015-1214-4.

Jardine, J., Relph, S., Magee, L.A., von Dadelszen, P. *et al.* (2020). Maternity services in the UK during the COVID-19 pandemic: A national survey of modifications to standard care. *BJOG: International Journal of Obstetrics and Gynaecology*. https://doi.org/10.1111/1471-0528.16547.

6  Tinkle, B., Castori, M., Berglund, B., Cohen, H. *et al.* (2017). Hypermobile Ehlers-Danlos syndrome (a.k.a. Ehlers-Danlos syndrome type III and Ehlers-Danlos syndrome hypermobility type): Clinical description and natural history. *American Journal of Medical Genetics Part C: Seminars in Medical Genetics*, 175(1), pp.48–69.

7  Tinkle, B., Castori, M., Berglund, B., Cohen, H. *et al.* (2017). Hypermobile Ehlers-Danlos syndrome (a.k.a. Ehlers-Danlos syndrome type III and Ehlers-Danlos syndrome hypermobility type): Clinical description and natural history. *American Journal of Medical Genetics Part C: Seminars in Medical Genetics*, 175(1), pp.48–69.

Edimo, C.O., Wajsberg, J.R., Wong, S., Nahmias, Z.P. and Riley, B.A. (2021). The dermatological aspects of hEDS in women. *International Journal of Women's Dermatology*. https://doi.org/10.1016/j.ijwd.2021.01.020.

8  Blagowidow, N. (2019). Gynecologic and obstetric issues in EDS and HSD [Video file]. Ehlers-Danlos Society. Accessed on 07/02/2023 at https://youtu.be/uFMbOzktWVE.

9  Roma, N.Z.H., Essa, R.M., Rashwan, Z.I. and Ahmed, A.H. (2023). Effect of dry heat application on perineal pain and episiotomy wound healing among primipara women. *Obstetrics and Gynecology International*. https://doi.org/10.1155/2023/9572354.

Kaur, N., Kaur Rana, A. and Suri, V. (2013). Effect Of dry heat versus moist heat on episiotomy pain and wound heating. *Nursing and Midwifery Research Journal*. https://doi.org/10.33698/nrf0150.

10  NHS (2020). Episiotomy and Perineal Tears. Accessed on 07/02/2023 at www.nhs.uk/pregnancy/labour-and-birth/what-happens/episiotomy-and-perineal-tears.

11  Carmichael, A. (2013). What patients say works for vulvodynia [Blog post]. 23andMe. Accessed on 07/02/2023 at https://blog.23andme.com/articles/what-patients-say-works-for-vulvodynia.

12  Glayzer, J.E., McFarlin, B.L., Castori, M., Suarez, M.L. *et al.* (2021). High rate of dyspareunia and probable vulvodynia in Ehlers–Danlos syndromes and hypermobility spectrum disorders: An online survey. *American Journal of Medical Genetics Part C: Seminars in Medical Genetics*, 187(4), pp.599–608.

13  Glayzer, J.E., McFarlin, B.L., Castori, M., Suarez, M.L. *et al.* (2021). High rate of dyspareunia and probable vulvodynia in Ehlers–Danlos syndromes and hypermobility spectrum disorders: An online survey. *American Journal of Medical Genetics Part C: Seminars in Medical Genetics*, 187(4), pp.599–608.

Morin, M., Binik, Y.M., Bourbonnais, D., Khalifé, S., Ouellet, S. and Bergeron, S. (2017). Heightened pelvic floor muscle tone and altered contractility in women with provoked vestibulodynia. *Journal of Sexual Medicine*, 14(4), pp.592–600.

14  Arunkalaivanan, A.S., Morrison, A., Jha, S. and Blann, A. (2009). Prevalence of urinary and faecal incontinence among female members of the Hypermobility Syndrome Association (HMSA). *Journal of Obstetrics and Gynaecology*, 29(2), pp.126–128.

Gilliam, E., Hoffman, J.D. and Yeh, G. (2020). Urogenital and pelvic complications in the Ehlers-Danlos syndromes and associated hypermobility spectrum disorders: A scoping review. *Clinical Genetics*, 97(1), pp.168–178.

15  Parry, J. (2021). Physiotherapy for adults with hypermobile Ehlers-Danlos syndrome and hypermobility spectrum disorders. Ehlers-Danlos Support UK. Accessed on 12/04/2023 at www.ehlers-danlos.org/information/physiotherapy-for-adults-with-hypermobile-ehlers-danlos-syndrome-and-hypermobility-spectrum-disorders.

16  Kazeminia, M., Rajati, F. and Rajati, M. (2022). The effect of pelvic floor muscle-strengthening exercises on low back pain: A systematic review and meta-analysis on randomized clinical trials. *Neurological Sciences: Official Journal of the Italian Neurological Society and of the Italian Society of Clinical Neurophysiology*. https://doi.org/10.1007/s10072-022-06430-z.

17  Cao, D., Rao, L., Yuan, J., Zhang, D. and Lu, B. (2022). Prevalence and risk factors of overt postpartum urinary retention among primiparous women after vaginal delivery: A case-control study. *BMC Pregnancy and Childbirth*. https://doi.org/10.1186/s12884-021-04369-1.

18  Nelson, A.D., Mouchli, M.A., Valentin, N., Deyle, D. *et al.* (2015). Ehlers Danlos syndrome and gastrointestinal manifestations: A 20-year experience at Mayo Clinic. *Neurogastroenterology and Motility*, 27(11), pp.1657–1666.

Arunkalaivanan, A.S., Morrison, A., Jha, S. and Blann, A. (2009). Prevalence of urinary and faecal incontinence among female members of the Hypermobility Syndrome Association (HMSA). *Journal of Obstetrics and Gynaecology*, 29(2), pp.126–128.

19  Lotfy Mohamed El Sayed, S. (2021). Effect of uterine massage and emptying of the urinary bladder on alleviation of afterpains among mothers in the immediate postpartum period. *International Journal of Africa Nursing Sciences*, 15, 100327.

20  Turawa, E.B., Musekiwa, A. and Rohwer, A.C. (2020). Interventions for preventing postpartum constipation. *Cochrane Database of Systematic Reviews*. https://doi.org/10.1002/14651858.cd011625.pub3.

21  Patel, R., Appannagari, A. and Whang, P.G. (2008). Coccydynia. *Current Reviews in Musculoskeletal Medicine*. https://doi.org/10.1007/s12178-008-9028-1.

22  Sabharwal, A. and Stocks, G. (2011). Postpartum headache: Diagnosis and management. *Continuing Education in Anaesthesia Critical Care and Pain*, 11(5), pp.181–185.

23  Do, T., Diamond, S., Green, C. and Warren, M. (2021). Nutritional implications of patients with dysautonomia and hypermobility syndromes. *Current Nutrition Reports*, 10(4), pp.324–333.

24  Hamonet, C., Delarue, M., Lefevre, J., Rottembourg, J. and Zeitoun, J. (2021). Ehlers-Danlos syndrome (EDS): A common and often disregarded cause of serious gastrointestinal complications in children and adults. *Scholarly Journal of Otolaryngology*. https://doi.org/10.32474/SJO.2021.07.000256.

25  Boushra, M. and Rathbun, K.M. (2021). Postpartum headache. In *Statpearls*. Treasure Island, FL: Statpearl Publishing. Accessed on 11/04/2023 at www.ncbi.nlm.nih.gov/books/NBK537101

26 Levy, A.R., Nnam, M., Gudesblatt, M. and Riley B. (2020). An investigation of headaches in hypermobile Ehlers-Danlos syndrome. *Annals of Psychiatry and Clinical Neuroscience*, 3(3), 1034.

27 Bendik, E.M., Tinkle, B.T., Al-shuik, E., Levin, L. *et al.* (2011). Joint hypermobility syndrome: A common clinical disorder associated with migraine in women. *Cephalalgia*, 31(5), pp.603–613.

28 Schievink, W.I., Gordon, O.K. and Tourje, J. (2004). Connective tissue disorders with spontaneous spinal cerebrospinal fluid leaks and intracranial hypotension: A prospective study. *Neurosurgery*, 54(1), pp.65–71.

Reinstein, E., Pariani, M., Bannykh, S., Rimoin, D.L. and Schievink, W.I. (2012). Connective tissue spectrum abnormalities associated with spontaneous cerebrospinal fluid leaks: A prospective study. *European Journal of Human Genetics*, 21(4), pp.386–390.

29 Goyal, V. and Srinivasan, M. (2010). Don't hold your breath. *Journal of General Internal Medicine*, 26(3), p.345.

Mokri, B. (2002). Spontaneous CSF leaks mimicking benign exertional headaches. *Cephalalgia*, 22(10), pp.780–783.

30 Arevalo-Rodriguez, I., Ciapponi, A., Roqué i Figuls, M., Muñoz, L. and Bonfill Cosp, X. (2016). Posture and fluids for preventing post-dural puncture headache. *Cochrane Database of Systematic Reviews*. https://doi.org/10.1002/14651858.cd009199.pub3.

31 Royal College of Obstetricians and Gynaecologists (RCOG) (2015). Reducing the Risk of Venous Thromboembolism during Pregnancy and the Puerperium. Green-top Guideline No. 37a. Accessed on 11/04/2023 at www.rcog.org.uk/media/qejfhcaj/gtg-37a.pdf.

32 Sultan, A.A., West, J., Tata, L.J., Fleming, K.M., Nelson-Piercy, C. and Grainge, M.J. (2011). Risk of first venous thromboembolism in and around pregnancy: A population-based cohort study. *British Journal of Haematology*, 156(3), pp.366–373.

33 Park, J.E., Park, Y. and Yuk, J.-S. (2021). Incidence of and risk factors for thromboembolism during pregnancy and postpartum: A 10-year nationwide population-based study. *Taiwanese Journal of Obstetrics and Gynecology*, 60(1), pp.103–110.

34 Castori, M., Morlino, S., Celletti, C., Ghibellini, G. *et al.* (2013). Re-writing the natural history of pain and related symptoms in the joint hypermobility syndrome/Ehlers-Danlos syndrome, hypermobility type. *American Journal of Medical Genetics Part A*, 161(12), pp.2989–3004.

35 Wiesmann, T., Castori, M., Malfait, F. and Wulf, H. (2014). Recommendations for anesthesia and perioperative management in patients with Ehlers-Danlos syndrome(s). *Orphanet Journal of Rare Diseases*. https://doi.org/10.1186/s13023-014-0109-5.

36 Al-Naseem, A., Sallam, A., Choudhury, S. and Thachil, J. (2021). Iron deficiency without anaemia: A diagnosis that matters. *Clinical Medicine*, 21(2), pp.107–113.

37 Zijp, I.M., Korver, O. and Tijburg, L.B. (2000). Effect of tea and other dietary factors on iron absorption. *Critical Reviews in Food Science and Nutrition*, 40(5), pp.371–398.

38 Gupta, P. (2022). Menstrual cycle effects on sleep. *Clinical Journal of Obstetrics and Gynecology*, 5(2), pp.42–43.

39  Hakim, A., De Wandele, I., O'Callaghan, C., Pocinki, A. and Rowe, P. (2017). Chronic fatigue in Ehlers-Danlos syndrome – hypermobile type. *American Journal of Medical Genetics Part C: Seminars in Medical Genetics*, 175(1), pp.175–180.

Pocinki, A. (2019). Sleep disorders in Ehlers-Danlos and related syndromes: A panoply of paradoxes [Video file]. Bobby Jones Chiari & Syringomyelia Foundation. Accessed on 30/01/2023 at https://youtu.be/Tr6Iv8_NVOw.

40  McKenna, J.J. and McDade, T. (2005). Why babies should never sleep alone: A review of the co-sleeping controversy in relation to SIDS, bedsharing and breast feeding. *Paediatric Respiratory Reviews*, 6(2), pp.134–152.

Fleming, P.J. and Blair, P.S. (2015). Making informed choices on co-sleeping with your baby. *BMJ*. https://doi.org/10.1136/bmj.h563

UNICEF (2019). *Co-sleeping and SIDS*. Accessed on 12/04/2023 at www.unicef.org.uk/babyfriendly/wp-content/uploads/sites/2/2016/07/Co-sleeping-and-SIDS-A-Guide-for-Health-Professionals.pdf.

Basis: Baby Sleep Info Source (n.d.). Bed-Sharing and Breastfeeding. Accessed on 06/02/2023 at www.basisonline.org.uk/hcp-bed-sharing-and-breastfeeding.

Unicef (2016). *Bed Sharing, Infant Sleep and SIDS: Research on Infant Health*. The Baby Friendly Initiative. Accessed on 12/04/2023 at www.unicef.org.uk/babyfriendly/news-and-research/baby-friendly-research/infant-health-research/infant-health-research-bed-sharing-infant-sleep-and-sids.

41  Fitz-Desorgher, R. (2017). *Your Baby Skin to Skin*. Bath: White Ladder.

42  Hugon-Rodin, J., Lebègue, G., Becourt, S., Hamonet, C. and Gompel, A. (2016). Gynecologic symptoms and the influence on reproductive life in 386 women with hypermobility type Ehlers-Danlos syndrome: A cohort study. *Orphanet Journal of Rare Diseases*. https://doi.org/10.1186/s13023-016-0511-2.

43  Rosseland, L.A., Reme, S.E., Simonsen, T.B., Thoresen, M., Nielsen, C.S. and Gran, M.E. (2020). Are labor pain and birth experience associated with persistent pain and postpartum depression? A prospective cohort study. *Scandinavian Journal of Pain*, 20(3), pp.591–602.

44  Segal, N.A., Boyer, E.R., Teran-Yengle, P., Glass, N.A., Hillstrom, H.J. and Yack, H.J. (2013). Pregnancy leads to lasting changes in foot structure. *American Journal of Physical Medicine and Rehabilitation*, 92(3), pp.232–240.

45  Gluppe, S., Ellström Engh, M. and Kari, B. (2021). Women with diastasis recti abdominis might have weaker abdominal muscles and more abdominal pain, but no higher prevalence of pelvic floor disorders, low back and pelvic girdle pain than women without diastasis recti abdominis. *Physiotherapy*. https://doi.org/10.1016/j.physio.2021.01.008.

Depledge, J., McNair, P. and Ellis, R. (2021). Exercises, Tubigrip and taping: Can they reduce rectus abdominis diastasis measured three weeks post-partum? *Musculoskeletal Science and Practice*, 53, 102381.

Depledge, J., McNair, P. and Ellis, R. (2022). The effect of Tubigrip and a rigid belt on rectus abdominus diastasis immediately postpartum: A randomised clinical trial. *Musculoskeletal Science and Practice*, 63, 102712.

46  Carlson, H., Colbert, A., Frydl, J., Arnall, E., Elliot, M. and Carlson, N. (2010). Current options for nonsurgical management of carpal tunnel syndrome. *International Journal of Clinical Rheumatology*, 5(1), pp.129–142.

47  Dhiman, N.R., Das, B., Mohanty, C., Singh, O.P., Gyanpuri, V. and Raj, D. (2021). Myofascial release versus other soft tissue release techniques along superficial back line structures for improving flexibility in asymptomatic adults: A systematic review with meta-analysis. (2021). *Journal of Bodywork and Movement Therapies*. https://doi.org/10.1016/j.jbmt.2021.06.026.

Ingraham, P. (2021). Does fascia matter?: The 'Father of Fascia' is so over it. PainScience.com. Accessed on 21/02/2023 at www.painscience.com/articles/does-fascia-matter.php#sec_father.

National Institute for Health and Care Excellence (NICE) (2021). Chronic Pain (Primary and Secondary) in over 16s: Assessment of All Chronic Pain and Management of Chronic Primary Pain. NG193. Accessed on 12/04/2023 at www.ncbi.nlm.nih.gov/books/NBK569984.

48  Martín-Santos, R., Bulbena, A., Porta, M., Gago, J., Molina, L. and Duró, J.C. (1998). Association between joint hypermobility syndrome and panic disorder. *American Journal of Psychiatry*, 155(11), pp.1578–1583.

Murray, B., Yashar, B.M., Uhlmann, W.R., Clauw, D.J. and Petty, E.M. (2013). Ehlers-Danlos syndrome, hypermobility type: A characterization of the patients' lived experience. *American Journal of Medical Genetics Part A*, 161(12), pp.2981–2988.

49  Nakić Radoš, S. (2018). Anxiety during pregnancy and postpartum: Course, predictors and comorbidity with postpartum depression. *Acta Clinica Croatica*, 57(1), pp.39–51.

50  Śliwerski, A., Kossakowska, K., Jarecka, K., Świtalska, J. and Bielawska-Batorowicz, E. (2020). The effect of maternal depression on infant attachment: A systematic review. *International Journal of Environmental Research and Public Health*, 17(8), 2675.

51  Niermeyer, M., Ball, D., Green, M., Jensen, B. *et al.* (2021). Interoceptive attention regulation in Ehlers–Danlos syndromes: Associations between pain and psychiatric symptom severity. *Translational Behavioral Medicine*, 11(10), pp.1923–1930.

52  Huang, L., Zhao, Y., Qiang, C. and Fan, B. (2018). Is cognitive behavioral therapy a better choice for women with postnatal depression? A systematic review and meta-analysis. *PLoS ONE*, 13(10), p.e0205243.

Milgrom, J., Gemmill, A.W., Ericksen, J., Burrows, G., Buist, A. and Reece, J. (2015). Treatment of postnatal depression with cognitive behavioural therapy, sertraline and combination therapy: A randomised controlled trial. *Australian and New Zealand Journal of Psychiatry*, 49(3), pp.236–245.

53  Bulut, S. and Gümüşsoy M., B. (2020). Postpartum depression and cognitive behavioral therapy from face to face group sessions to online group sessions. *Psychology and Psychotherapy: Research Study*, 4(2), pp.1–5.

54  Sheydaei, H., Ghasemzadeh, A., Lashkari, A. and Ghorbani Kajani, P. (2017). The effectiveness of mindfulness training on reducing the symptoms of postpartum depression. *Electronic Physician*, 9(7), pp.4753–4758.

55  Bear, K.A., Barber, C.C. and Medvedev, O.N. (2022). The impact of a mindfulness app on postnatal distress. *Mindfulness*. https://doi.org/10.1007/s12671-022-01992-7.

56  NHS (2021). NHS Talking Therapies. Accessed on 12/04/2023 at www.nhs.uk/mental-health/talking-therapies-medicine-treatments/talking-therapies-and-counselling/nhs-talking-therapies.

57  Hugon-Rodin, J., Lebègue, G., Becourt, S., Hamonet, C. and Gompel, A. (2016). Gynecologic symptoms and the influence on reproductive life in 386 women with hypermobility type Ehlers-Danlos syndrome: A cohort study. *Orphanet Journal of Rare Diseases*. https://doi.org/10.1186/s13023-016-0511-2.

58  Uvnäs Moberg, K. and Prime, D.K. (2013). Oxytocin effects in mothers and infants during breastfeeding. *Infant*. Accessed on 12/04/2023 at www.infantjournal.co.uk/pdf/inf_054_ers.pdf.

McKenna, J.J. (2014). Night waking among breastfeeding mothers and infants: Conflict, congruence or both? *Evolution, Medicine, and Public Health*, 2014(1), pp.40–47.

59  Śliwerski, A., Kossakowska, K., Jarecka, K., Świtalska, J. and Bielawska-Batorowicz, E. (2020). The effect of maternal depression on infant attachment: A systematic review. *International Journal of Environmental Research and Public Health*, 17(8), 2675.

Pope, C.J. and Mazmanian, D. (2016). Breastfeeding and postpartum depression: An overview and methodological recommendations for future research. *Depression Research and Treatment*. https://doi.org/10.1155/2016/4765310.

60  Śliwerski, A., Kossakowska, K., Jarecka, K., Świtalska, J. and Bielawska-Batorowicz, E. (2020). The effect of maternal depression on infant attachment: A systematic review. *International Journal of Environmental Research and Public Health*, 17(8), 2675.

61  Francis, J. and Dickton, D.D. (2022). Considerations for lactation with Ehlers-Danlos syndrome: A narrative review. *International Breastfeeding Journal*. https://doi.org/10.1186/s13006-021-00442-9.

62  Gazit, Y., Jacob, G. and Grahame, R. (2016). Ehlers–Danlos syndrome—hypermobility type: A much neglected multisystemic disorder. *Rambam Maimonides Medical Journal*, 7(4), e0034.

63  Drugs and Lactation Database (LactMed®) (2006). Nifedipine. Accessed on 12/04/2023 at www.ncbi.nlm.nih.gov/books/NBK501047.

64  Anderson, J.E., Held, N. and Wright, K. (2004). Raynaud's phenomenon of the nipple: A treatable cause of painful breastfeeding. *Pediatrics*, 113(4), pp.e360–e364.

65  The Breastfeeding Network (2019). Cracked Nipples and Moist Wound Healing. Accessed on 12/04/2023 at www.breastfeedingnetwork.org.uk/moist-wound-healing.

66  Francis, J. and Dickton, D.D. (2022). Considerations for lactation with Ehlers-Danlos syndrome: A narrative review. *International Breastfeeding Journal*. https://doi.org/10.1186/s13006-021-00442-9.

67  International BreastFeeding Centre (2020). Breastfeeding and Medications. Accessed on 12/04/2023 at https://ibconline.ca/information-sheets/breastfeeding-and-medications.

68  The Breastfeeding Network (2022). Drugs Factsheets. Accessed on 12/04/2023 at www.breastfeedingnetwork.org.uk/drugs-factsheets.

69  Breastfeeding and Medication (n.d.). Home [Facebook page]. Accessed on 06/02/2023 at www.facebook.com/breastfeedingandmedication.

70  Hale, T.W. (2021). *Hale's Medications & Mothers' Milk 2021: A Manual of Lactational Pharmacology*. New York: Springer Publishing Company.

71  The Breastfeeding Network (2021). Codeine and Breastfeeding. Accessed on 12/04/2023 at www.breastfeedingnetwork.org.uk/codeine.

72  Moran, F. (2021). Statement on the use of opioids in pain management of the Ehlers-Danlos syndromes and hypermobility spectrum disorders. Ehlers Danlos Society. Accessed on 31/01/2023 at www.ehlers-danlos.com/statement-on-the-use-of-opioids-in-pain-management-of-the-ehlers-danlos-syndromes-and-hypermobility-spectrum-disorders.

Epstein, M., Song, B., Yeh, P., Nguyen, D. and Harrell, J. (n.d.). *Ehlers Danlos Syndrome: A Retrospective Review of the Current Treatment Options in Pain Management.* Accessed on 31/01/2023 at www.texaspain.org/assets/2019AnnualMeeting/EpsteinEDS_Retrospective_Review.pdf.

Bachmutsky, I., Wei, X.P., Kish, E. and Yackle, K. (2020). Opioids depress breathing through two small brainstem sites. *eLife*, 9, p.e52694.

73  Suomi, S.J. (1995). Influence of Attachment Theory on Ethological Studies of Biobehavioral Development in Nonhuman Primates. In S. Goldberg, R. Muir and J. Kerr (eds) *Attachment Theory: Social, Developmental, and Clinical Perspectives* (pp. 185–201). Hillsdale, NJ: Analytic.

74  Gravel-Miguel, C., Cristiani, E., Hodgkins, J., Orr, C.M. *et al.* (2022). The ornaments of the Arma Veirana Early Mesolithic infant burial. *Journal of Archaeological Method and Theory.* https://doi.org/10.1007/s10816-022-09573-7.

75  Anon. (n.d.). Baby Sling Safety: The T.I.C.K.S Rule for Safe Babywearing. Accessed on 12/04/2023 at http://babyslingsafety.co.uk.

76  Sling Libraries Network. (n.d.). Find a Sling Library Near You. Accessed on 23/02/2023 at https://ukslinglibraries.wordpress.com.

77  Jackson, A. (2008). Time to review newborn skincare. *Infant*, 4(5), pp.168–171.

78  Bell, L. and Pearce, G. (2021). Parents' experiences of children's health care for hypermobile Ehlers–Danlos syndrome and hypermobility spectrum disorders. *Children's Health Care.* https://doi.org/10.1080/02739615.2021.1960165.

79  Demmler, J.C., Atkinson, M.D., Reinhold, E.J., Choy, E., Lyons, R.A. and Brophy, S.T. (2019). Diagnosed prevalence of Ehlers-Danlos syndrome and hypermobility spectrum disorder in Wales, UK: A national electronic cohort study and case-control comparison. *BMJ Open*, 9(11), e031365.

80  Casanova, E.L., Baeza-Velasco, C., Buchanan, C.B. and Casanova, M.F. (2020). The relationship between autism and Ehlers-Danlos syndromes/hypermobility spectrum disorders. *Journal of Personalized Medicine.* https://doi.org/10.3390/jpm10040260.

Kindgren, E., Quiñones Perez, A. and Knez, R. (2021). Prevalence of ADHD and autism spectrum disorder in children with hypermobility spectrum disorders or hypermobile Ehlers-Danlos syndrome: A retrospective study. *Neuropsychiatric Disease and Treatment*, 17, pp.379–388.

81  Murray, K.J. and Woo, P. (2001). Benign joint hypermobility in childhood. *Rheumatology*, 40(5), pp.489–491.

82  Adib, N., Davies, K., Grahame, R., Woo, P. and Murray, K.J. (2005). Joint hypermobility syndrome in childhood. A not so benign multisystem disorder? *Rheumatology*, 44(6), pp.744–750.

Jelsma, L.D., Geuze, R.H., Klerks, M.H., Niemeijer, A.S. and Smits-Engelsman, B.C. (2013). The relationship between joint mobility and motor performance in children with and without the diagnosis of developmental coordination disorder. *BMC Pediatrics.* https://doi.org/10.1186/1471-2431-13-35.

Williams, D.J., Jaggi, A. and Douglas, T. (2020). The association between crawling as a first mode of mobilisation and the presentation of atraumatic shoulder instability: A retrospective cohort study. *Shoulder and Elbow*. https://doi.org/10.1177/1758573220968485.

83  Lamari, M.M., Lamari, N.M., Araujo-Filho, G.M., Medeiros, M.P., Pugliesi Marques, V.R. and Pavarino, É.C. (2022). Psychosocial and motor characteristics of patients with hypermobility. *Frontiers in Psychiatry*. https://doi.org/10.3389/fpsyt.2021.787822.

84  Smith, A. (2018). Police tore baby from mother's arms when condition was mistaken for abuse. *Metro*. Accessed on 12/04/2023 at https://metro.co.uk/2018/01/12/police-tore-baby-from-mothers-arms-when-genetic-condition-was-mistaken-for-abuse-7223696.

85  Smith, A. (2018). Police tore baby from mother's arms when condition was mistaken for abuse. *Metro*. Accessed on 12/04/2023 at https://metro.co.uk/2018/01/12/police-tore-baby-from-mothers-arms-when-genetic-condition-was-mistaken-for-abuse-7223696

Ehlers Danlos Society (2023). Child Protection, EDS, and HSD. Accessed on 27/02/2023 at www.ehlers-danlos.com/child-protection-and-eds.

86  Lai, N.M., Ahmad Kamar, A., Choo, Y.M., Kong, J.Y. and Ngim, C.F. (2017). Fluid supplementation for neonatal unconjugated hyperbilirubinaemia. *Cochrane Database of Systematic Reviews*. https://doi.org/10.1002/14651858.cd011891.pub2.

87  Kawchuk, G.N., Fryer, J., Jaremko, J.L., Zeng, H., Rowe, L. and Thompson, R. (2015). Real-time visualization of joint cavitation. *PLoS ONE*, 10(4), e0119470.

88  De Pellegrin, M., Damia, C.M., Marcucci, L. and Moharamzadeh, D. (2021). Double diapering ineffectiveness in avoiding adduction and extension in newborns hips. *Children*, 8(3), p.179.

89  Celletti, C., Castori, M., La Torre, G., Grammatico, P., Morico, G. and Camerota, F. (2011). Reassessment of oral frenula in Ehlers-Danlos syndrome: A study of 32 patients with the hypermobility type. *American Journal of Medical Genetics Part A*, 155(12), pp.3157–3159.

Conti, R., Zanchi, C. and Barbi, E. (2021). A floppy infant without lingual frenulum and kyphoscoliosis: Ehlers Danlos syndrome case report. *Italian Journal of Pediatrics*, 47. https://doi.org/10.1186/s13052-021-00984-y.

90  Fitz-Desorgher, R. (2016). All tied up. Tongue tie and its implications for breastfeeding. *Practising Midwife*, 6(1), pp.20–22. Accessed on 28/02/2023 at https://pubmed.ncbi.nlm.nih.gov/12599967.

91  Castori, M., Dordoni, C., Morlino, S., Sperduti, I. *et al.* (2015). Spectrum of mucocutaneous manifestations in 277 patients with joint hypermobility syndrome/Ehlers-Danlos syndrome, hypermobility type. *American Journal of Medical Genetics Part C: Seminars in Medical Genetics*, 169(1), pp.43–53.

92  Griffiths, D.M. (2004). Do tongue ties affect breastfeeding? *Journal of Human Lactation*, 20(4), pp.409–414.

Berry, J., Griffiths, M. and Westcott, C. (2012). A double-blind, randomized, controlled trial of tongue-tie division and its immediate effect on breastfeeding. *Breastfeeding Medicine*, 7(3), pp.189–193.

93  Association of Tongue-Tie Practitioners (n.d.). Home. Accessed on 12/04/2023 at www.tongue-tie.org.uk.

94   Fitz-Desorgher, R. (2017). *Your Baby Skin to Skin*. Bath: White Ladder.

Fardig, J. (1980). A comparison of skin-to-skin contact and radiant heaters in promoting neonatal thermoregulation. *Journal of Nurse-Midwifery*, 25(1), pp.19–28.

Widström, A., Brimdyr, K., Svensson, K., Cadwell, K. and Nissen, E. (2019). Skin-to-skin contact the first hour after birth, underlying implications and clinical practice. *Acta Paediatrica*, 108(7), pp.1192–1204.

95   Fitz-Desorgher, R. (2017). *Your Baby Skin to Skin*. Bath: White Ladder.

Savino, F., Clara Grassino, E., Guidi, C., Oggero, R., Silvestro, L. and Miniero, R. (2006). Ghrelin and motilin concentration in colicky infants. *Acta Paediatrica*, 95(6), pp.738–741.

Weissbluth, L. and Weissbluth, M. (1992). Infant colic: The effect of serotonin and melatonin circadian rhythms on the intestinal smooth muscle. *Medical Hypotheses*, 39(2), pp.164–167.

96   Kalliomaki, M. (2001). Short report: Extent of fussing and colic type crying preceding atopic disease. *Archives of Disease in Childhood*, 84(4), pp.349–350.

97   Seneviratne, S.L., Maitland, A. and Afrin, L. (2017). Mast cell disorders in Ehlers-Danlos syndrome. *American Journal of Medical Genetics Part C: Seminars in Medical Genetics*, 175(1), pp.226–236.

98   Hong, Y.R. and Park, J.S. (2012). Impact of attachment, temperament and parenting on human development. *Korean Journal of Pediatrics*, 55(12), pp.449–454.